PRAISE FOR
SUPERHEALTH

"Dr. Pratt's *SuperHealth* is a practical and easy guide to keep you young, healthy, and in shape. Dr. Pratt has done a super job in compiling all the latest health research and making it palatable to mainstream Americans."
—Ann Louise Gittleman, *New York Times* bestselling author of *The Fat Flush Plan* and *Before the Change*

"If you have been searching for fresh and innovative ways to slim down and shape up, feel better and prevent disease, *SuperHealth* will rock your world. It is a research-based, no-nonsense guide that offers simple ways to significantly enhance your life. Steve Pratt provides the key; unlock the door to a new you."
—Daniel A. Nadeau, M.D., author of *The Color Code: A Revolutionary Eating Plan for Optimum Health*

- Find out why adding the right fruit to your diet mimics calorie restriction and makes you lose weight even if you don't eat less
- Learn how to use food and exercise to turn off bad genes and turn on the good ones
- Discover the foods and nutrients that keep your hearing, vision, and other senses as young as when you were in your twenties
- See why detoxing your home and your car can reverse and even prevent disease
- Know which foods keep toxins out of your body
- Understand what blood sugar levels and waist circumference tell you about your future

Also by Steven Pratt, M.D.

The SuperFoods Rx Diet:
Lose Weight with the Power of SuperNutrients
by Wendy Bazilian, Steven Pratt, and Kathy Matthews

SuperFoods HealthStyle:
Simple Changes to Get the Most Out of Life for the
Rest of Your Life by Steven Pratt and Kathy Matthews

SuperFoods Rx:
Fourteen Foods That Will Change Your Life
by Steven Pratt and Kathy Matthews

SuperHealth

6 Simple Steps,
6 Easy Weeks,
1 Longer, Healthier Life

Steven Pratt, M.D.

WITH SHARYN KOLBERG

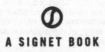

A SIGNET BOOK

SIGNET
Published by New American Library, a division of
Penguin Group (USA) Inc., 375 Hudson Street,
New York, New York 10014, USA
Penguin Group (Canada), 90 Eglinton Avenue East, Suite 700, Toronto,
Ontario M4P 2Y3, Canada (a division of Pearson Penguin Canada Inc.)
Penguin Books Ltd., 80 Strand, London WC2R 0RL, England
Penguin Ireland, 25 St. Stephen's Green, Dublin 2,
Ireland (a division of Penguin Books Ltd.)
Penguin Group (Australia), 250 Camberwell Road, Camberwell, Victoria 3124,
Australia (a division of Pearson Australia Group Pty. Ltd.)
Penguin Books India Pvt. Ltd., 11 Community Centre, Panchsheel Park,
New Delhi - 110 017, India
Penguin Group (NZ), 67 Apollo Drive, Rosedale, North Shore 0632,
New Zealand (a division of Pearson New Zealand Ltd.)
Penguin Books (South Africa) (Pty.) Ltd., 24 Sturdee Avenue,
Rosebank, Johannesburg 2196, South Africa

Penguin Books Ltd., Registered Offices:
80 Strand, London WC2R 0RL, England

Published by Signet, an imprint of New American Library, a division of Penguin
Group (USA) Inc. Previously published in a Dutton edition.

First Signet Printing, January 2010
10 9 8 7

Ⓡ REGISTERED TRADEMARK—MARCA REGISTRADA

Printed in the United States of America

PUBLISHER'S NOTE
Every effort has been made to ensure that the information contained in this
book is complete and accurate. However, neither the publisher nor the author
is engaged in rendering professional advice or services to the individual reader.
The ideas, procedures, and suggestions contained in this book are not intended
as a substitute for consulting with your physician. All matters regarding your
health require medical supervision. Neither the author nor the publisher shall
be liable or responsible for any loss or damage allegedly arising from any information or suggestion in this book. The opinions expressed in this book represent the personal views of the author and not of the publisher.

The recipes contained in this book are to be followed exactly as written. The
publisher is not responsible for your specific health or allergy needs that may
require medical supervision. The publisher is not responsible for any adverse
reactions to the recipes contained in this book.

The publisher does not have any control over and does not assume any
responsibility for author or third-party Web sites or their content.

In loving memory of my mom and dad,
who continually stressed that an ounce of prevention
is worth more than a pound of cure.

Acknowledgments

I would like to thank my wife, Gunilla, for her patience, love and support, organizational skills, and yummy recipes, all of which have played an essential part in completing this book and keeping me in the Super-Health "zone." All my kids, Mike and his wife, Diane, Tyler, Torey, Brian, Jennifer, Grant, and Marlaina, have seen me working away on weekends to put this book together, and I really appreciate their encouraging words. A special thanks to Torey, for once again she has done a great job of providing me with an incredible amount of research material for *SuperHealth*. Thank you to my office staff, Maurya Troiano and Carol Henry, and to all my patients for putting up with my often very hectic schedule. A special thanks to the world's best librarian, Kimberly Baker, for her unbelievable ability to find the answer to just about any question regarding research, outcomes, and so on related to *SuperHealth*.

As always, the SuperFoods Rx partners, Ray Sphire, David Stern, and Hugh Greenway, have provided enthusiastic support and constant encouragement for this project.

Thank you, Dr. Mimi Guarneri, Dr. Robert Bonakdar, and the rest of the Scripps Center for Integrative Medicine crew, Dr. Victor Sierpina and his wife, Michelle, Dr. Howard Hunt, and Dr. Stewart Richer, for setting such a great example for all health-care professionals by pushing forward with techniques and research aimed at preventing many of the chronic diseases facing us in the twenty-first century.

Thanks to Deborah Szekely, eighty-something-year-old youngster and founder of the Golden Door and Rancho La Puerta spas, for setting the bar high for all future "oldsters." And to the folks at Cal-a-Vie Spa for resetting my clock after I finished the manuscript of this book.

Sharyn Kolberg has been unbelievable in her ability to turn science into prose with humor, while at the same time proving to be a real pro in the "putting a book together" department. Sharyn, I cannot thank you enough!

Amy Hertz, you are the most involved, professional, hands-on in a good way editor! Keep up your marvelous work, and thanks to your assistant, Melissa Miller, who is learning fast from one of the great editors—you. Amy and Melissa, you are two of the most competent and caring people I've ever met! And thanks to David Vigliano and Dan Ambrosio for making this book a reality.

Lastly, thanks to the late Martha Kruger (my good friend and patient who giggled her way to 101 and continually reminded me of the health benefits of laughter and optimism), and my friend Bob Denton, who, in the late 1980s, showed me a book by Jean Carper discussing the many health benefits associated with individual foods.

Publisher's Note

Neither the publisher nor the author is engaged in rendering professional advice or services to the individual reader. The ideas, procedures, and suggestions contained in this book are not intended as a substitute for consulting with your physician. All matters regarding your health require medical supervision. Neither the author nor the publisher shall be liable or responsible for any loss or damage allegedly arising from any information or suggestion in this book.

The recipes contained in this book are to be followed exactly as written. The publisher is not responsible for your specific health or allergy needs that may require medical supervision. The publisher is not responsible for any adverse reactions to the recipes contained in this book.

Contents

Part II: The SuperHealth Reference Guide

Part III: Appendix and Bibliography

The SuperHealth Program

The
Supercash
Program

1

Genesis

When I was in my early forties, I had a revelation. For years my son Mike and I had races up our driveway. I beat him almost every time. Then one day I realized that my seventeen-year-old son could run up our driveway more times, and each time faster than I could, no matter how hard I tried and how hard I worked out. I was shocked. I couldn't keep up.

I couldn't keep up, but I did not give up. Instead I changed my goal. I was not going to try to outrun my son. I realized that it's not possible to run as fast when you are forty-plus as you did when you were twenty. I also realized that even if I couldn't run like Mike, I could at least run up the driveway more times and at a faster clip than any of my contemporaries.

What I needed was a plan, a blueprint for aging well in order to ensure that I would be as healthy as I could possibly be until the day I died. I wanted to live, in good health and good spirits, to see my kids turn one hundred. That made me think about my mom, who lived into her nineties. She was always a great inspiration to me, and she knew more about nutrition than anyone I've ever met. She had no degree in the subject, never went to school for it. She did read voraciously and so got some of her knowledge from books, but a lot of what she knew was from information passed down from her mother, from her intuition, and from her common sense.

She was a powerhouse of knowledge, which she was vigilant about passing on to her children. We had no sugary snacks around the house. Instead we had huge bowls of shelled sunflower seeds (for the vitamin E, I now know). There was no sitting around doing nothing. There was "go outside and run around the block." There was a constant reminder to stand up straight, shoulders back, head up. She knew so much more than doctors or even health food experts knew back then. Before I began to study nutrition myself, when patients would ask me a food-related question, I'd have them call my mom. She always knew the answer. You'll meet my mom periodically as you read through this book—she's gone now, but her tips and lessons live on.

I have taken those lessons and combined her knowledge with the latest cutting-edge, research-based, scientific information to design the program I put together for this book. What I came up with was SuperHealth, a six-week, six-step program that gives you the best foods to eat to promote health and prevent disease. It's a simple blueprint for adding exercise into your life, getting more sleep, and reducing stress.

If today's amazing scientific breakthroughs tell us anything about aging, it's that we have more opportunities than ever before to stave off debilitating diseases, maintain an active lifestyle, and take advantage of our ever-increasing average life spans. Every day researchers are making extraordinary discoveries about aging, about what happens to our bodies as we get older, and about what steps we can take to prolong a vigorous, meaningful, and healthy life.

Do these scientific breakthroughs guarantee a life that is vital to the very end? They're not as futuristic as many people believe. Cutting-edge science is telling us what we need to do to keep up with the technical advances that are allowing us to live many more years—and the answers are not very technical at all. In fact,

they do not require thousands of dollars of investment
or expensive equipment or exotic curatives from the
mountains of the Himalayas. Science is now telling us
it's the synergy of the right foods, the right nutrients,
and the right lifestyle choices that provide us with "bio-
insurance": the steps you can take today to ensure a
longer, healthier, more vital future.

IT'S EASIER THAN YOU THINK

Although *SuperHealth* started out as a plan for extending my own life span, my patients really inspired me to
write this book. I always talk to my patients, no matter
what their current age, about living longer and dying
happier. We have intense conversations about living to
be one hundred. And I'm flabbergasted every time a patient says to me, "But, Dr. Pratt, I don't want to live that
long." I ask them why, and I always get the same answer:
"Because by the time I'm one hundred," they say, "I'll
be in a nursing home, I'll be impotent and incontinent.
I'll look terrible and I won't be able to think, I won't be
able to see, I won't be able to hear." This is the assumption that most of my patients have: that you have to
spend the last years of your life in such a state of ill
health that you don't want to be alive in the first place.

SuperHealth was written to blow that assumption
away, to tell you that it is not a foregone conclusion that
you have to be sick and in ill health for the last part of
your life. And that's not just me speaking; there's a huge
amount of scientific data in peer-reviewed published
studies that show that an infirm old age doesn't have to
be the case, that you don't have to get cancer, heart disease, Alzheimer's disease, or any of the chronic illnesses
of aging. You certainly don't have to spend the last
quarter of your life in such a state of ill health that you
don't want to live much longer than sixty, seventy, or
eighty years old.

And what you'll discover in this book is that living to
a vital, intact old age is a lot easier and more fun than

you may have thought. There are in fact six easy steps you can take that cover many of the aspects people are worried about. Their brain, their eyes, their heart, their strength, their stamina. They want to be able to prevent the six major causes of premature death: lung, colon, breast, and prostate cancer, heart disease, and stroke. If you knock those out of the equation, there's not a lot left out there that's going to get you. The goal is to flame out at the finish line and have your death certificate read "Died of old age—with a smile on his (or her) face." That's just the way Mom went.

What I most want you to know is that it's easy and fun to achieve SuperHealth. You don't have to become a new person or change your entire lifestyle or give up everything you like. Watching your weight, for instance, which really involves watching your waist, which in turn helps control your blood sugar, is important because it turns out that controlling your blood sugar may be the key to living a longer and healthier life. Yes, you may need to lose weight—but not as much as you think. You can add years to your life via the "10 percent solution," which means losing just 10 percent of your excess body weight. You can use the simple techniques you'll find here to help you keep your brain sharp and functioning as you get older, to get the sleep you need, and to reduce the stress in your life. You'll discover simple steps you can take to preserve your senses as you age, and to look good while you're doing it.

You'll learn that physical activity may be what keeps you young. When I talk to my patients about exercise, many of them have the same reaction. "But, doc," they say, "I'm not a jock or a super athlete." The good news is you don't have to be. All you have to do is get yourself moving. A recent study from the *Journal of the American Medical Association* showed that people who burned an extra 287 calories a day had a 32 percent lower risk of mortality as compared to those who moved less, with an astounding 67 percent lower risk for the most active (in burning calories) individuals. Best of all, the authors concluded, "Simply expending energy through ANY activity may influence survival in older adults." We were born to move, and we die prematurely if we don't. What this study shows is that you don't have to be a jock to get some movement into your life. You don't have to think of exercise in the traditional sense. All household chores count as exercise. Go for a walk. Mess around in the garden. If you're going to talk on the telephone, stand up and move around while you're talking. Even people who fidget burn more calories and potentially live longer than those who don't. Anything that burns a calorie is going to extend your life and your health span.

You'll also learn that one of the keys to getting old successfully and living a long life is to remain optimistic and look at aging with a "glass is half full" attitude, even if there's nothing but moisture left on the bottom. We don't have control over the twists and turns that life presents to us, but every second of every single day we have control over how we react to those events. We don't have to be happy all the time or pretend that bad things don't happen. This book is about how to become an expert in life and in living, and how to get the biggest bang for your SuperHealth buck. I am not promising eternal life on earth, but I am saying that if you follow the six steps you will markedly improve your chances of getting into the SuperHealth zone. Once there, you will love it, and in fact you will love the journey you take to get there—I do promise you'll find it fun and rewarding and challenging at the same time!

SUPERHEALTH: YOUR OWN LONGEVITY CLINIC

As much as people tell me they don't want to live to be one hundred, their assertion is belied by the fact that longevity clinics are sprouting like proverbial weeds all over the country. Their popularity tells me that people actually are interested in living longer. What people don't want is the decline in physical function that occurs with aging and represents the early stage of a continuum of other important adverse outcomes such as the "dreaded nursing home." Although the rate of disability from 1982 to 2004 declined in the United States (three cheers for us), the absolute number of disabled older adults is projected to increase as the population ages over the next two decades. So who can blame us for wanting a longevity clinic to solve our problems? Unfortunately, many of these clinics rely on untested drugs and supplements to fulfill the public's desire to take the Ponce de León approach, looking for the magical fountain of youth or an instant anti-aging pill. We all know it doesn't work that way.

SuperHealth gives you a much better shot at living longer and better, not with potentially dangerous injections, exotic herbs we've never heard of before, or fancy fad diets that come and go, but with simple solutions like making sure we have enough essential nutrients in our diets, which we can get from everyday foods like blueberries, salmon, spinach, and tea.

That's what SuperHealth is all about—taking small, simple steps that together add up to a huge leap forward in the way we approach health care, both individually and as a society. Western medicine is so focused on treating disease that prevention is often ignored. That is partly because there's very little incentive to prevent disease. For the most part, the health-care industry doesn't make money by preventing disease; it makes money by treating it. It makes my blood boil when I see headlines like the one that appeared in the *San Diego Union-Tribune* in February 2008: "Annual Health Care Spending Expected to Double by 2017." Overall health-care spending in 2017 is estimated to increase to $4.3 trillion—about 20 percent of the gross national product. If that happens, you won't have to worry about your disease state; you won't even have enough money for your Depends! It's part of my obligation as a doctor, as an American, and as a citizen of the world to find ways of keeping us from going broke because of health-care costs. How about spending some of that money on bringing fresh vegetables into the school system, on restoring physical education programs where they have been reduced or eliminated? Parents are so concerned with having their kids go up to their rooms to study; maybe it's time we made room for family activities that get everyone burning some calories.

The information in this book is the best preventive measure you can take against premature aging and ill health. It's all in one easy, accessible place for you. Too many times you have to go from specialist to specialist or from book to book to get the information you want and need in order to get the full health picture. You don't have to do that anymore, because it's all right here for you, laid out in a week-by-week, easy-to-follow plan you can start today and continue for the rest of your life.

We may not all get to see our kids turn one hundred, but the SuperHealth program can help add years to your life, and, even better, extend your health span to closely match your life span. It's never too early or too late to get the benefits from SuperHealth's six easy steps. It's simple: Science has now validated Mom's advice. It turns out that Mom really did know best.

2

The SuperHealth
Promise and Getting Started

You're never too old to start feeling young, nor too young to keep yourself from aging prematurely. Super-Health is not just about extending your life, but about extending the quality of your life by tweaking your habits to feel good for the rest of your life. And who doesn't want to feel good every day?

My belief is that no one should feel old until they're one hundred. By then you've earned it. In the meantime there's no reason you can't be sixty-five, seventy-five, or eighty-five and active, healthy, and vibrant, without loss of vision, without hearing aids, without walkers, and without twenty-five different medications you can never remember to take.

Is aging inevitable? Of course it is. We can slow it down and make it more pleasant, but it will happen to all of us. It doesn't have to be something we dread or fear, though. The more we learn about how to take care of our bodies, aging though they are, the better our older years will be, because although aging is inevitable, the diseases and maladies of aging need not be.

SuperHealth does not mean being SuperHuman— it's not about trying to be perfect. It's about taking advantage of the homespun knowledge that has been passed down to us for generations about what's good for us to eat and do on a daily basis and melding it into the most up-to-date facts science has to offer about how nutrition works at the cellular level. It is about learning to utilize numerous resources easily available to you (in your local supermarket, your neighborhood health food store, your kitchen cabinet, or your own backyard) in order to obtain and maintain the best possible health throughout your lifetime.

It's about making small changes in your life that add up to a longer, healthier life. I know you can make them. These are changes I've made in my life, and I wouldn't ask you to do anything I wouldn't do. I'm asking you to add some healthy, nutritious (and tasty) foods to your diet. You're probably eating most of them already; you might just have to pump up the volume on some of them. I'm asking you to move a little more than you do right now. If you want to go to the gym, good for you, but if not, there are plenty of things you can do while you watch TV or listen to the radio.

None of this is complicated, costly, or difficult to implement. These are easy steps to follow. I'll tell you why each one is important to your health and show you how following this simple plan will help you:

- Live longer
- Retrieve that glow of good health that makes you look and feel younger
- Pump up your energy level no matter what your age or size
- Regain your excitement for life
- Keep your mind sharp and functioning at its best as you age
- Resist the chronic illnesses that often come with aging
- Feel good for the rest of your life

Maybe you think your family history is a hurdle you can't get over. SuperHealth can show you how, by making small changes in your diet and behavior, you can help influence your genetic destiny and live healthier and happier than you ever imagined. You won't grow old gracefully—you'll grow old glowing, fit, and more energetic than your TV-watching, video-gaming children and grandchildren.

CHEATING THE DISEASES OF MODERN MAN

No quest to achieve SuperHealth would be complete—or effective—without mentioning the major causes of death in the United States (and around the world) and how to prevent them. Here are some disturbing facts about the top six killers in the United States today: heart attack, stroke, and the four leading cancers—prostate, breast, lung, and colorectal.

- Myocardial infarction (MI), commonly known as a heart attack, is the leading cause of death among Americans—both men and women. In 2008 it was estimated that 565,000 people in the United States would have a heart attack for the first time and another 300,000 would have a repeat MI. Statistics also show that within one year of a heart attack 18 percent of men and 23 percent of women will die. Within five years after an attack about 33 percent of men and 43 percent of women will die.
- Stroke is the third leading cause of death after heart disease and cancer, and it is the number one cause of disability. Every year about 700,000 people in the United States have a stroke. On average someone in the United States has a stroke every forty-five seconds. According to the World Health Organization, about 15 million people worldwide per year fall victim to a stroke. About 5 million of those will die and another 5 million will be left permanently disabled (see pages 323–29 for a list of steps you can take to avoid cardiovascular disease).
- When the subject is cancer, you come across a variety of sobering statistics. For instance, the Amer-

ican Cancer Society (ACS) estimated that in 2008 there would be 745,180 men and 692,000 women diagnosed with cancer in this country. Cancers of the prostate and breast were the most frequently diagnosed cancers in men and women, respectively, followed by lung and colorectal cancers in both men and women. The ACS also estimated that 294,120 men and 271,530 women would die of these diseases. According to the Centers for Disease Control and Prevention, one in two men and one in three women in the United States will develop some form of cancer during their lives.

The bad news is that the cancer death rate in 2005 was only slightly lower than the death rate in 1950, while death rates for other major chronic diseases (like heart disease and stroke) decreased substantially during that period. The good news is that the survival rates for all cancers combined and for certain site-specific cancers have improved significantly since the 1970s, due in part to earlier detection and advances in treatment. Survival rates markedly increased for cancers of the prostate, breast, colon, and rectum and for leukemia. With new treatment techniques and increased utilization of screening, there is hope for even greater improvements in the not-too-distant future.

The good news is that it is estimated that up to 80 percent of colon, breast, and prostate cancer cases and one-third of all cancer cases may be influenced by diet and associated lifestyle factors. (See pages 329–36 for a list of steps you can take to avoid these cancers.)

The best news here for both cardiac and cancer patients is also the worst news. It is the diet and lifestyle of the Western world that is putting more of us at risk. Living in the twenty-first century can be tricky business for us human beings. On the one hand, those of us who live in first-world countries are often surrounded by abundance and convenience. We have plenty to eat. We have ultrafast and (for the most part) safe means of transport. We have ease of communication. We have myriad ways to keep ourselves entertained. We have a technically advanced medical system that has helped millions of us survive diseases that would have been death sentences even twenty-five years ago. We have a lot to be thankful for.

On the other hand, we have "abundanced" ourselves into deep, deep trouble. Our ease of transportation and communication has made it possible to socialize without much physical effort. We can talk, we can text, we can e-mail; we can make our travel arrangements and drive, fly, or travel by train, and the only body parts that get a workout are our fingers as they whisk across the keyboard.

As to having plenty to eat—here's where the old saying "too much of a good thing" comes into play. Or maybe in this situation it's too much of a not-so-good thing, as it's not really that we eat too much (although many of us eat more than we need); the problem is more that we eat too many foods that are not very good for us. Many of the foods we eat are in fact downright unhealthy. So while we are rushing to take advantage of every medical technology that allows our bodies to last longer, we're actually aging ourselves prematurely by not treating our bodies with the care and feeding they deserve.

That's what SuperHealth is all about: taking care of yourself, plain and simple. And it is, in many ways, a lot simpler than we think. This is what I've tried to emphasize in all my books—getting healthy (and staying that way) isn't difficult. Does it take some effort? Of course it does. Everything worthwhile takes some effort. But what Super-Health takes mostly is *thought*—thinking about how you live your life and what's important to you. SuperHealth takes some attitude adjustment. Would you rather watch reality television for the next several years or live more of your own life in the real world? And SuperHealth means making decisions. Do you want to eat more junk food or get more out of life? By making some simple alterations (how hard is it to add blueberries, green tea, or honey to your menu?) in your diet and lifestyle and exchanging good habits for bad, you can make positive, long-lasting changes in your life.

What the SuperHealth program does is stack the odds in your favor. For instance, we know that people who eat the most fruits and vegetables are half as likely to develop cancer as those who eat the least amount. Eat more vegetables, cut your odds for getting cancer by 50 percent. Simple. In another example, studies have shown that women who are physically active have about half the risk of heart disease compared to those who do not exercise. The best news is that walking turns out to be a good way to cut the risk—and it doesn't even have to be fast-paced. All you have to do is walk one hour a week. That works out to less than ten minutes a day. Walk for ten minutes a day and cut the odds of heart disease in half. Simple. Then there's sleep. Researchers have found that people who consistently sleep less than seven hours a night had a nearly 25 percent increased risk of death compared to those who did get their seven hours in. Get more sleep, give yourself a better chance of living longer. Simple.

These simple solutions work because they actually address the underlying causes of the major diseases of our times (cardiovascular disease, cancer, diabetes), which include high blood sugar, high blood pressure, systemic inflammation, and oxidative stress (too many free radicals and not enough antioxidants to neutralize them, which in turn can lead to inflammation and the onset of multiple diseases such as cardiovascular disease, cancer, and macular degeneration). When we eat our veggies, get off our duffs, and get our zzz's, we're providing the kind of environment in which our cells were meant to thrive. We're allowing our bodies to work the way they were programmed to work and function at their highest capacities to add vital, energetic years to our lives.

HOW THE SUPERHEALTH PROGRAM WORKS

There are six steps in the SuperHealth program. Each of the successive chapters is one more step in the program. These steps are:

- **Step 1: Control Your Genes Through Omega-3 Fatty Acids and Resveratrol**—We all know that many aspects of our health are inherited from our parents, grandparents, and ancestors. But science now tells us that we are not doomed to live out a genetic destiny that will send us to the grave with our mother's heart disease or our father's cancer. The exciting, emerging field of nutrigenomics is introducing us to new ways to use food and lifestyle choices to suppress our "bad" genes and express the "good" ones that help prevent disease, counter environmental toxins, and increase longevity factors.

- **Step 2: Become an Environmentalist and Detox Your Body**—You're only as healthy as the natural world in which you live. You don't have to be a fanatic to improve your own health and the health of the planet. There are a number of simple things you can do to "green" your environment and keep your body, your home, and your workplace free of pollutants and toxins. Personal awareness of the world around us is not only essential to the future of humankind; it's one of the best ways to stay alive and healthy in that world.

- **Step 3: Watch Your Waistline—Burn Those Calories**—Two easy measurements—your blood sugar level and your waist circumference—can be the single most significant guidelines to your ongoing health, vigor, and longevity. One of the best ways to assure those two measurements are where you want them to be is through physical exercise. There's no simpler message in the health field lexicon than "use it or lose it." We are genetically programmed to move—historically you either get going or you're a goner. We've got to use our bodies to keep our health. The benefits of exercise have been proven to go far beyond controlling your weight—from boosting your immune system to preventing and/or slowing the progression of diseases like cancer, degenerative eye disease, and dementia. In fact, exercise can improve every single aspect of your life—especially as you age. Super-Health lets you know you don't have to be an elite athlete to get the benefits of physical activity; you can ramp up your exercise without going to the gym. Small increments—walking for an additional ten or twenty minutes a day—can make a world of difference.

- **Step 4: Control Inflammation**—Inflammation is the underlying factor of virtually all diseases encountered in the twenty-first century. There are many scientifically valid, natural ways to control this phenomenon before you "burn up" and flame out. Find out which nutrients are best for reducing inflammation and how sleep, reducing stress, and exercise are essential for tamping down the fire inside in order to reduce the risk of heart disease, Alzheimer's disease, cancer, diabetes, and many other ailments.

- **Step 5: Keep Up Appearances**—It's not just vanity anymore—the science "behind the looking glass" tells us that paying attention to our skin, joints, and muscles both optimizes appearance and provides benefits that are far more than skin deep.

- **Step 6: Preserve Your Senses**—One of the greatest fears about aging is loss of cognitive function; however, proper dietary and lifestyle choices can virtually assure us that we will be able to count those candles as we mature. The second greatest fear is that as we grow older we will no longer be able to use our senses to appreciate the world around us. There's no denying that our bodies change as we age. Our eyesight weakens, our hearing diminishes, even our taste buds are not what they used to be.

Not only can this detract from our pleasure in life; it can affect our health as well. Luckily we can take the simple steps outlined in Chapter 8 to preserve and sharpen our senses as we age.

The SuperHealth program is designed to build on itself week after week. For instance, in Step 1 in Chapter 3 you'll be introduced to the concept of how diet and lifestyle can influence your genes. In that chapter you'll find the SuperFoods that are particularly good for "turning on" good genes and suppressing bad ones. A weekly chart will give you a visual aid to show you how you can add these foods into your life, and a shopping list at the end of the chapter will give you brand-name suggestions for how to stock your SuperHealth kitchen for the week. In each successive chapter you'll find the list of Super-Foods particularly good for that week's step, the weekly food (and exercise) charts, and the weekly shopping list. Some foods may be repeated in more than one step; that is because all SuperFoods have multiple benefits. If you're eating spinach for your eyesight, that's great—because it will also help you turn on your "good" genes, reduce inflammation, lose weight. . . . You get the idea. So don't think that you're limited each week to only the Su-perFoods in that week's list. You can mix and match whichever foods please you most. The weekly foods and charts are just a simple way to ease you into making healthier choices. By the end of the book you will have been introduced to each of the twenty-five SuperFoods and fifteen SuperNutrients deemed the best for optimal health.

GETTING STARTED

Each of the weeks in the program focuses on a specific, select group of foods, and just as I want you to see the food lists as launch pads, I also want you to be sure to remember the basics. Some of the weekly lists focus on fruits, some on proteins, some on veggies, but under-

SuperHealth Food Pyramid

Compare and contrast the weekly lists with this Pyramid to make sure you're getting your daily *balance*. What are you getting? What are you missing? Sometimes the lists will cover the Pyramid, sometimes they'll have holes. Look here to make sure you fill in the blanks.

Fruits: 3–5 servings daily; try to find room for berries every day

Vegetables: Unlimited (minimum 5–7 servings); dark, leafy greens are the best

Whole Grain and Whole Grain Fiber: 5–7 servings of Whole Grains *or* 10–20 grams of Whole Grain Fiber; sample a variety of whole grains— cereals, noodles/pasta, breads

Protein: *Animal Protein:* 1–2 servings six days per week of skinless poultry breast/fish; may include 4 oz of grass-fed lean red meat once a week. Go meatless at least once per week.

Vegetarian Protein: 1–3 servings daily of legumes, lentils, soy (i.e., tempeh, tofu), egg whites, egg (1 per day maximum)

Skeletal Strength: 1–3 servings daily of non- or low-fat dairy, tofu, soy, fortified soy milk, fortified OJ, fish with bones (i.e., sardines, canned salmon), shellfish, dark, leafy greens

Daily Protein Consumption Guide:

If you're under 65 and . . .
You weigh under 125 lbs try to get *45 grams of protein*
You weigh 125–150 lbs try to get *55 grams of protein*
You weigh 150–200 lbs try to get *73 grams of protein*

If you're over 65 . . .
Divide your weight in pounds by 2 to estimate the grams of protein you need.

Healthy Fats: 1–2 servings daily of nuts, seeds, avocado, and 1–2 servings of extra-virgin olive oil, canola oil, soybean oil, peanut oil

Serving Guide

Fruits: 1 baseball

Vegetables: 1½ baseballs

Beans: ½ cup cooked

Animal Protein: 1 deck of cards fish/ poultry and 1 deck of cards red meat
Or
Vegetarian Protein: 1 baseball

Skeletal Strength: 1 baseball for solids or 1 8-oz glass for liquids

Healthy Fats: 1 golf ball to ½ baseball solids or 1 shot glass healthy oils

Healthy Fun: 1 golf ball

Spice It Up: Add spices to taste daily.

Healthy Fun: 100 calories daily of dark chocolate, butter, buckwheat honey, sweets, or refined bread and grains neath it all we still need to be sure we're getting a little bit of everything every day. That's why, in addition to each week's SuperFood list, I want you to follow the **SuperHealth Food Pyramid** on page 19 to be sure that you're hitting all the food groups each day, every week. Think of the weekly lists as a bonus paycheck on top of your daily nutritional earnings.

In each of the chapters of this book you will find specific steps you can take to improve your chances of living the healthy, vibrant life you want. You'll also find profiles of some of my patients who are living examples of SuperHealth at work. They've been kind enough to share their stories with me, and I now share them with you.

In the end, this book is really about synergy. The overriding theme is that the sum total of all the steps gives you a far bigger bang for your healthy buck than taking one or two steps and skipping all the others. Better to do some than none, of course, but if you want to optimize your chances of living a long, active, vital life, if you want to be the best that you can be for the longest amount of time, then following all six steps will help you get there. If you get plenty of rest but eat a junk-food diet, you lower your chances. If you eat well but never get up off the couch, you lower your chances. If you exercise daily without relieving a stress-filled life, you lower your chances. And if you do everything else "right" but sleep only two hours a night, you're going to be in big trouble. Nobody's perfect. But if you crowd out your bad habits with good ones, if you fill your day with healthy and enjoyable habits instead, you won't have the time or inclination to go back to your old behavior patterns. Everybody can feel great and attain SuperHealth with these six easy steps.

◆ MEET MRS. FELLOWS ◆

Ninety-seven and Going Strong

Ask Thyra Fellows the secret to long life, and you get a hearty laugh in response. "I don't have any secrets," she says. "It's probably my strong German heritage." But then, after she thinks about it for a while, a few things do come to mind. There's her diet, for instance. "I was probably more inclined to eat fruits and vegetables than many other people I know." Growing up in Toledo, Ohio, Fellows always had a garden where she grew beans and tomatoes. But her knowledge of food didn't start, she says, until she was married and learned to cook for herself and her family. "I think it was easier for me to eat well, because when I was a child we didn't have all the things on the grocery shelves they have today. All of that stuff that is so bad for you. I always tried to eat a balanced diet."

Mrs. Fellows also says she learned to listen to her body. When she was a child, she would often sit and eat a lemon while reading a book. "Oranges were not readily available in Ohio then, and when they were, they were very expensive. So I ate lemons. I didn't know it at the time, but my body was craving citrus. Eating lemons gave me what I needed."

Mrs. Fellows will also tell you that she's been active all her life. She played golf and tennis and loved to ice skate and roller skate. But more than that, she's walked a great deal. "I'm ninety-seven years old and when I had my bone density tested a few years ago, they had to do it twice because they didn't believe it. It was +2 (and -1 is considered normal)! When I was young—and remember, this was almost one hundred years ago—we didn't have a car. We lived within walking distance of my school and of going downtown when I went to work. Even after I grew up, I just kept on walking."

Of course, nobody is perfect, and Mrs. Fellows does admit to a bad habit or two. She smoked cigarettes for about six years in the 1950s, but hated being "addicted to something that had control of me." So she kicked the habit. And to this day she likes sweets a little bit more than she should. "I love chocolate, and I've eaten a lot of chocolate bars in my life. Now everybody says chocolate is good for you. I guess I knew it all along."

3

Step 1: Control Your Genes Through Omega-3 Fatty Acids and Resveratrol

For your basics, see the SuperHealth Food Pyramid, page 19 (for your bonus, see below)

Week 1 Omega-3 SuperFoods:

Wild salmon
Spinach
Walnuts

Soy and soybean oil
Flaxseed

Week 1 Resveratrol SuperFoods:

Peanuts/Peanut butter
Purple grapes
Purple grape juice

Blueberries
Cranberries/Cranberry juice
Red wine

Two friends go on the same weight-loss diet. One loses fifty pounds, the other twelve. Two other people begin to make dietary changes to lower their blood pressure. One is successful; the other ends up needing medication. Nutritionally these two pairs were consuming identical diets, yet they reacted differently. Why? Because losing weight and controlling blood pressure, along with most common illnesses, such as diabetes, heart disease, many cancers, and several psychiatric diseases, involve a combination of both environmental—outside—and genetic—inside—factors.

In the best of all possible worlds it would be routine for you to visit your doctor for DNA testing, and then a week or two later be handed a chart of the best foods and lifestyle choices for you and the specific vitamins and supplements you need in exactly the right doses to perfectly balance your nutrient needs. Each and every one of us would have an individually designed nutrition plan to help prevent and potentially treat or cure disease.

We aren't there yet, but we are on our way.

There is an emerging field of science known as nutrigenomics, or nutritional genomics, which is focused on how various nutrients in foods and supplements may influence the way your genes work (or don't work). Researchers are looking at how various components in food help to access a cell's DNA library to then signal a gene to produce proteins that make the cell work. In other words, scientists are trying to discover how we can turn on "good" genes and turn off "bad" genes by eating specific gene-nurturing foods.

This is not a new pursuit. Hippocrates, the renowned Greek physician and the father of modern medicine, recognized that nutrition played an important role in health. And since ancient times, traditional Chinese and Indian Ayurvedic medicine have both devised systems that address individual problems through the use of a variety of herbs and foods to treat specific diseases.

But now modern science has given us a tool humankind never had before, and that is the completion of the human genome sequence, which is giving us an unprecedented amount of knowledge concerning human genetics. All humans are 99.9 percent identical at the gene sequence level. The .1 percent variation produces the difference in phenotype: the observable traits or characteristics of an individual; for example, hair color, weight, or the susceptibility to disease or health. It is this variation that causes, for instance, some people to be able to lower their blood pressure through dietary changes while others need drugs, and why some people are more susceptible to inflammatory diseases, or gastrointestinal problems, or asthma. The next step is to begin to understand the very complex relationship between our genes, our lifestyle, and the many food components that are known to influence the expression of genes in humans. This is the "promise" for the future: learning how to personalize this relationship and take advantage of it on an individual basis.

LIFE IS LIKE A POKER GAME

It's not always the player with the best cards who wins the game. You're not doomed just because you've been dealt a bad genetic hand. Nor are you necessarily safe if you've been dealt a royal flush of good genes. What allows you to hedge your bets is how you play those cards. Every time you make a healthy choice of diet and exercise, you up the ante and start raking in the chips (and I don't mean potato, either!).

When we think of our genetic inheritance, we usually think that it's set in stone, so to speak. Some of it is. If we inherit brown eyes and brown locks, we can disguise them with contact lenses and hair coloring, but we can't change what we got in the mix from our parents. If, on the other hand, we inherit a tendency to develop arthritis, there are things we can do using the foods we eat to stop (or at least slow down) the "arthritis genes" from expressing what would otherwise be their destiny.

The whole promise and premise is that food components can act on the human genome (the genetic information contained in our DNA), either directly or indirectly to alter the expression of genes, and that diet could potentially compensate for or accentuate effects of genetic polymorphisms (the differences in DNA sequence among individuals). The consequences of diet are dependent on the balance of health and disease states and on an individual's genetic background, the idea being that you are not doomed if you got a dose of bad genes from Mom and/or Dad, because you can use SuperFoods and lifestyle choices to help control the expression of your genetic heritage.

NUTRITION VERSUS DISEASE

Our bodies are in a constant state of shifting balance between health and potential disease. The complex interplay of genes, the environment, and lifestyle choices (such as exercise and sleep), which includes diet, is what tips the balance in one direction or the other. When the balance tips too far in the direction of an unhealthy nutritional environment, we are subject to disease. In our modern world we tend to intervene after the fact; that is, we treat signs and symptoms of disease after they have already occurred. By doing so we ignore the underlying conditions that cause major diseases, such as:

- the imbalance of omega-3/omega-6 fatty acids by not getting enough healthy fats (from fish, nuts, and seeds, for example), too much grain-fed red meat, and too many processed foods rich in only omega-6 fatty acids
- lack of phytonutrients, vitamins, and minerals from not having enough unprocessed and unrefined whole foods in our diet
- lack of fiber from not eating enough whole grains, fruits, and vegetables
- lack of vitamin D from not getting enough sun and not eating enough vitamin D–fortified foods
- high sodium/low potassium from too many processed foods and a diminished intake of fruits, vegetables, and legumes (such as peas, beans, and lentils)
- lack of exercise, which historically has been the primary way we have burned calories and has been one of our body's key longevity-enhancing modalities
- lack of sleep (adequate sleep is the most overlooked health-promoting strategy)

It is these underlying conditions that cause these diseases:

- cardiovascular disease
- cancer
- diabetes and other diseases related to obesity
- inflammatory diseases such as rheumatoid arthritis, irritable bowel syndrome, and Crohn's disease

If you look closely at the list of underlying conditions, one thing pops right out at you: They are all reversible. We can add more healthy fats to our diet by eating wild salmon, nuts, seeds, and extra-virgin olive oil; more important phytonutrients (nonvitamin, nonmineral nutrients that have health benefits when consumed) by eating whole grains; and more fiber by eating fruits, vegetables, and legumes. We can get our body moving and then give it the rest it needs. We may not be able to eliminate disease altogether, but we can protect our bodies with the armature that SuperHealth provides. And we can do it in increments following the SuperHealth program in an easy, step-by-step manner that leads to a longer, healthier life.

SUPERHEALTH BEGINS

Scientists are now discovering that not all of the food we eat is metabolized for energy. A small percentage of dietary chemicals become ligands—molecules that bind to proteins involved in "turning on" certain genes. It appears that some nutrients can turn on genes that head us in the direction of good health, while others can lead us down the path of chronic illness.

We begin the SuperHealth program with two Super-Nutrients that are critical for turning on our good genes: omega-3 fatty acids and resveratrol.

Omega-3s and the Best Sources of Omega-3s

Omega-3 fatty acids are found in fish and certain plant sources such as green leafy vegetables, walnuts, and flaxseed that, among other benefits, act to lower the levels of triglycerides (fats in our bodies we get from eating animal products and saturated fat) in the blood, lower systolic and diastolic blood pressure and heart rate, and decrease the production of inflammatory chemicals produced by our bodies.

You will note that the SuperFoods listed throughout the book have "sidekicks" as well. These are foods with similar nutrient properties that can be used as alternative choices in your weekly plans.

For the "I Hate Fish" Crowd

There are some people who just can't stomach the taste of fish. If you find yourself in that category, you should be taking a fish oil supplement daily. Even if you are a fish lover, there may be days when you're not getting enough omega-3s, so I recommend that everyone take EPA/DHA supplements twice daily with meals (500 to 1000 milligrams a day for adult women, 1000 to 2000 milligrams a day for adult men). Keep the bottle in the fridge once it's been opened. My favorite brands include Trader Joe's Darwin's Omega-3 Fatty Acid Dietary Supplements; MaxiVision Omega-3 Formula; MaxiTears Dry Eye Formula (888-290-6294); Life Extension Super Omega-3 (800-544-4440); Nordic Naturals Ultimate Omega (www.nordicnaturals.com); Alaskan Sockeye Salmon Oil (www.vitalchoice.com); Lovaza (by prescription only; ask your doctor about it); the soft-gel capsule found in the SuperFoods Rx daily dose packets (www.superfoodsrx.com); and DHA from algae (such as Nature's Way EFAGold Neuromins Plant Source Microalgae Oil, 100 milligrams DHA, (www.naturesway.com).

FISH SOURCES (EPA/DHA): WILD SALMON

Recommended amount: 3 to 4 ounces (1 deck of cards), two to four times a week

Sidekicks: Alaskan/northern halibut, canned chunk light or albacore tuna, mackerel, sardines, farmed trout, herring, sea bass, oysters, and clams (farmed or wild)

PLANT SOURCES (ALPHA-LINOLENIC ACID [ALA]): SPINACH

Recommended amount: 1 cup steamed (1 baseball) or 2 cups raw most days

Sidekicks: other green leafies with ALA include purslane and collard greens

Here's my favorite way of eating spinach—I eat this salad almost every day, sometimes twice a day, partly because of all its great health benefits but mostly because it's so delicious.

❖ SuperHealth Spinach Salad

1 cup spinach torn into bite-size pieces
1 cup chopped romaine lettuce
¼ cup shredded red cabbage
½ cup sliced red bell pepper (or orange, yellow, or green bell pepper)
½ tomato, chopped
¼ cup chickpeas; if canned, rinse well (the water they are packed in can be quite salty)
½ cup grated carrot
¼ avocado, cubed
2 tablespoons extra-virgin olive oil
1 teaspoon balsamic vinegar

Combine the spinach, lettuce, cabbage, red pepper, tomato, chickpeas, carrot, and avocado in a bowl. In a separate bowl, whisk together the oil and vinegar. Toss the dressing with the salad just before serving.

Add a sprinkle of ground peppercorns, a handful of your favorite chopped fresh herbs, 1 tablespoon Parmigiano-Reggiano, or 2 tablespoons roasted nuts or seeds. This quantity is for one person, but you can easily scale up the ingredients to serve more.

PLANT SOURCES (ALPHA-LINOLENIC ACID [ALA]): WALNUTS

Recommended amount: 1 handful (1 layer spread across your palm), five times weekly

Sidekicks: other nuts and seeds with ALA include pumpkin seeds, pecans, and pistachios

I like all kinds of nuts, so I usually rotate the types of nuts I eat. I keep several containers of nuts in the refrigerator at work and at home. Once the package is open, nuts should be refrigerated so the oil in them does not go rancid. This also gives you portion control—if they stay in the fridge rather than in a bowl on the coffee table, you can grab one handful and leave it at that. If they're out in the open, you'll be tempted to keep eating as you read or watch TV. The exception is walnuts because nuts in the shell don't go bad, and having to use a nutcracker to open each one keeps you from eating too many. I also prefer raw nuts rather than dry-roasted nuts because the heat can have some adverse effects on the fat, making them a source of unhealthy fats, just what your genes don't need.

Consumer Alert: In the United States purslane is considered a weed. In Europe it is a popular salad green. It's so good for you that I would place it on par with spinach. If I could find it here in California I'd eat it every day.

Your best bet for finding purslane is at a local farmers' market (it's in season from April through November). If you can't find it there, ask your grocer to find a source, or go to a well-informed nursery; they may either grow it or be able to get some for you to grow yourself. It's a great source of omega-3s.

PLANT SOURCES (ALPHA-LINOLENIC ACID [ALA]):
SOY

Recommended amount: 10 to 15 grams of soy protein a day (see label for protein per serving)

Sources: soybeans, tofu, omega-3 fortified Silk soymilk, soy nuts

I usually get my soy from a cup of soymilk in my cereal every morning; you can also use it for making smoothies, pancakes, muffins, and cakes. I often use soymilk in Dr. Steve's Hot Chocolate (see recipe, page 280). Many people (especially vegetarians) use tofu as a protein source, as it can be baked, broiled, or grilled and is good in stir-fries and soups.

PLANT SOURCES (ALPHA-LINOLENIC ACID [ALA]):
FLAXSEED

Recommended amount: 2 tablespoons a day (2 tablespoons = 1 shot glass)

Sidekick: wheat germ

You can buy whole flaxseeds and grind them yourself (ground flaxseeds are easiest to digest), and they are best ground immediately before use. Preground flaxseed is not quite as good but is an option if you're sure to keep it in the fridge. You can find ground flaxseed in many supermarkets and most health food stores. For a tasty treat or dessert, sprinkle a teaspoon or two over yogurt and berries.

PLANT SOURCES (ALPHA-LINOLENIC ACID [ALA]):
SOYBEAN OIL

Recommended amount: up to 2 tablespoons a day (1 shot glass)

Sidekicks: canola oil

Soybean oil is best used in salad dressing or cooking.

Other Sources of Omega-3s

DHA Eggs: If you're going to eat eggs, choose ones that are DHA-enriched (a good source is Eggland's Best; www.eggland.com). A recent study demonstrated that six DHA-enriched eggs a week supply a measurable bioavailable source of this healthy fat (if you have diabetes, check with your physician about how many eggs a week you should be consuming).

Other sources of omega-3s are Premium Dark Chocolate from the SuperFoods Kitchen (about 1.6 ounces, or half a bar a day) or Cocoa Tickles (about .75 ounce; www.cocoatickles.com), SuperFoods Kitchen Frozen Pizza (www.superfoodsrx.com), and A.C. LaRocco Frozen Pizza (www.aclarocco.com). One serving is one-third of a pizza.

Absolute musts: If there's only one omega-3-rich food you add for the week, or if you're traveling and can't control your diet, my recommendation is an EPA/DHA supplement (500 to 1000 milligrams a day for adult women and 1000 to 2000 milligrams a day for adult men).

Week 1: Omega-3 Daily Planner

The chart on page 32 is an example of how you can add omega-3s to your SuperHealth program. It shows you how to get more omega-3s into your diet—but it doesn't mean these are the only foods you should eat for the week. This is what I want to see you work into your diet so that you'll be able to turn off the bad genes and turn on the good genes. These are just suggestions—you can customize your planner from everything listed in this chapter, so feel free to mix and match foods and days to your heart's content (and health).

	Food Suggestion	**Daily Servings**
Day 1	Wild salmon	3–4 ounces (1 deck of cards)
	Spinach	1 cup steamed (1 baseball)
	Walnuts	1 handful (1 layer on your palm)
	Soymilk	2 cups (16 ounces)
	Flaxseed	2 tablespoons ground (1 shot glass)
Day 2	DHA eggs	2 eggs
	Spinach	2 cups raw (2 baseballs)
	Pecans	1 handful (1 layer on your palm)
	Tofu	½ cup raw tofu (½ baseball)
	Wheat germ	2 tablespoons (1 shot glass)
	Soybean oil	2 tablespoons (1 shot glass)
Day 3	Alaskan halibut	3–4 ounces (1 deck of cards)
	Spinach	1 cup steamed (1 baseball)
	Soymilk	2 cups (16 ounces)
	Flaxseed	2 tablespoons ground (1 shot glass)
Day 4	Pecans	1 handful (1 layer on your palm)
	Soymilk	2 cups (16 ounces)
Day 5	DHA eggs	2 eggs
	Collard greens	1 cup steamed (1 baseball)
	Pumpkin seeds	1 handful (1 layer on your palm)
	Tofu	½ cup raw tofu (½ tennis ball)
	Flaxseed	2 tablespoons ground (1 shot glass)
Day 6	Canned chunk light tuna	3–4 ounces (1 deck of cards)
	Soy nuts	1 handful (1 layer on your palm)
	Flaxseed	2 tablespoons ground (1 shot glass)
	Soybean oil	1 tablespoon (½ shot glass)
Day 7	DHA eggs	2 eggs
	Spinach	2 cups raw (2 baseballs)
	Walnuts	1 handful (1 layer on your palm)
	Soymilk	2 cups (16 ounces)
	Wheat germ	2 tablespoons (1 shot glass)
	Canola oil	1 tablespoon (½ shot glass)

OMEGA-3S AND YOUR GENES

The single most important step you can take to protect your genetic environment is to have the right ratio of omega-3 fatty acids to omega-6 fatty acids.

Both omega-3s and omega-6s are forms of essential fatty acids, and both are necessary for human health. Neither can be produced by the body; therefore, they must be obtained from the foods we eat. Omega-3s come from foods such as the ones listed above (such as wild salmon, ground flaxseed, green leafy vegetables), while omega-6s are found in whole grains, soy, corn and corn oil, pumpkin and sunflower seeds, cottonseed oil, safflower seed oil, nuts, grain-fed beef (don't be confused—some foods, such as soy and pumpkin seeds, have both omega-3s and omega-6s), and most processed foods, including most crackers, frozen foods, and packaged cakes and cookies. Unfortunately, processed foods such as white bread and white pasta contain an abundance of omega-6s, oftentimes hydrogenated. That means you are getting disease-causing trans fats. This is not where to get your omega-6s. If you do, the balance between omega-3s and omega-6s will be thrown off, tipping your body toward a pro-inflammatory state, which leads to cardiovascular disease, cancer, and in fact most causes of death related to modern man. Most of us get more omega-6s than we need, but from all the wrong places, such as too much vegetable oil and processed foods like white bread and white pasta, cookies, and crackers, turning on all the wrong genes.

Before all these processed foods were available, human beings managed to consume close to a 1:1 ratio of the two omegas. A healthy diet should consist of no more than two or three times more omega-6 fatty acids than omega-3 fatty acids, otherwise the abundance of omega-6s will turn on too many pro-inflammatory genes. The closer you are to a 1:1 ratio, the lower the likelihood of turning on disease-causing bad genes. However, most Americans don't eat a healthy diet. In our fast-food, convenience-oriented society, the typical American consumes roughly fifteen to twenty-five times more omega-6s than omega-3s because that's the ratio that comes in fast food and most packaged foods.

Here's one of the reasons for this imbalance: There are three major types of omega-3s—alpha-linolenic acid (ALA), eicosapentaenoic acid (EPA), and docosahexaenoic acid (DHA). Plant-based omega-3s (such as spinach, walnuts, flaxseed, and canola oil) contain ALA. When ALA enters the body, it is converted into EPA and DHA, which are the types found in marine fish oils and are more readily used by the body. There is a conversion rate of anywhere from 1 to 15 percent of ALA to EPA/DHA. But when you get beyond a 3:1 ratio of omega-6 to omega-3, that conversion rate goes way, way down (and it is low to begin with).

Because most Americans get most of their omega-3s from plants, not fish, it's extremely important to keep as high a conversion rate as possible. The more you get of this healthy fat, the more likely you are to express healthy genes and create an environment in your body in which it's tougher to develop cancer, heart disease, macular degeneration, obesity, cardiac arrhythmia (irregular heartbeat), and decreased mental function.

The expression of genetic information can be highly dependent on and regulated by the nutrients, micronutrients, and phytonutrients found in food. A diet in which the omega-3/omega-6 ratio is not balanced can alter gene-nutrient interactions, thereby increasing the risk of developing chronic disease like heart disease and cancer. SuperFoods and SuperNutrients, as well as healthy fat and healthy fat ratios, provide an environment in your body to optimize the expression of good genes and suppress the expression of bad genes.

VITAMIN D, THE SUPERLONGEVITY NUTRIENT

Vitamin D is the new SuperNutrient that might as well be called the new SuperLongevity Nutrient. In the past few years there's been an explosion of research on its far-reaching benefits for all age groups: It helps decrease blood sugar, it helps you maintain a healthy blood pressure, it helps decrease inflammation, it helps prevent the growth of abnormal, unwanted blood vessels as found in cancer and macular degeneration, it helps preserve muscle strength and function, it helps fortify calcium intake, it's great for your bone health. It helps maintain grip strength, protect against fibromyalgia, multiple sclerosis, and depression. It's an immune system booster, helps with cell growth, and, last but not least, it helps prevent colorectal, breast, prostate, pancreatic cancers, and death from melanoma or non-Hodgkin's lymphoma.

Recommended amount: Aim for consuming two foods daily containing vitamin D_2 or D_3 (all nonfortified vitamin D found in foods is vitamin D_3). In addition, expose skin (you make the choice of what parts) to sunlight for fifteen minutes at least three times a week, remembering that there is no vitamin D production from sunlight during the winter months in many parts of the world. Take a vitamin D_3 supplement daily, with teens and older adults aiming for 600 to 2000 IU of supplemental D_3 daily.

Stick to Salmon, Sunlight, and Supplements

To be sure that you're reaping the enormous benefits of vitamin D, here are a couple of tips I try to follow:

- Eat 3 to 4 ounces, or a deck of card's worth, of wild salmon (I like Alaskan wild salmon) at least twice a week.
- Get outside to get sunshine. Aim for fifteen minutes at least three times a week. Wear sunscreen and catch your rays before 10 a.m. and after 4 p.m. so that you get the benefits of the sun without too much UV.
- On top of that, I recommend taking 600 to 2000 IU of vitamin D supplements or drinking vitamin D–fortified milk or soymilk and orange juice.

Resveratrol and the Best Sources of Resveratrol

Resveratrol is a phytonutrient that is being researched for its anti-inflammatory and anti-aging abilities, as well as its potential cancer-fighting properties. In most cases it looks like it inhibits the expression of genes for these problems.

PEANUTS/PEANUT BUTTER

Recommended amount: For peanuts, 1 handful (1 layer on your palm), five times weekly; for peanut butter, 2 tablespoons a day (2 tablespoons = 1 walnut in a shell). The peanut skins are an especially great source for resveratrol.

PURPLE GRAPES

Recommended amount: 1 to 2 cups (1 to 2 baseballs), five to seven days a week. The resveratrol is in the grape skins.

PURPLE GRAPE JUICE

Recommended amount: 1 cup, divided into two ½ cups with meals daily

BLUEBERRIES

Recommended amount: 1 to 2 cups (1 to 2 baseballs) daily

CRANBERRIES/CRANBERRY JUICE

Recommended amount: ½ cup cranberries daily (½ baseball; buy frozen and mix with less bitter berries) or ½ cup cranberry juice (mix 100 percent pure cranberry juice with blueberry or Concord grape juice) daily

RED WINE

Recommended amount: For those of you who choose to drink; for women: one to three 4.5-ounce glasses a week; for men: two to six 4.5-ounce glasses a week.

Absolute musts: If there's only one resveratrol-rich food you add for the week, or if you're very busy or traveling and can't control your diet, my recommendation is ½ cup two times daily of 100 percent Concord grape juice (preferably juice that comes in a glass rather than a plastic container).

Week 1: Omega-3 and Resveratrol Daily Planner

The chart below is an example of how you can add resveratrol to your SuperHealth program. You can interchange any of these resveratrol choices for any other, with two exceptions: If you have more than one nut serving per day—for example walnuts for omega-3 and peanuts or peanut butter for resveratrol—you may want to adjust your calorie intake for the day. And stay within the recommended weekly guidelines for choosing red wine.

	Food Suggestion	Daily Servings
Day 1	Blueberries	1 cup (1 baseball)
Day 2	Purple grape juice	½ cup, twice a day
Day 3	Peanut butter	2 tablespoons (1 walnut in a shell)
Day 4	Red wine	one 4.5-ounce glass
Day 5	Blueberries	1 cup (1 baseball)
Day 6	Peanuts	1 handful (1 layer on your palm)
Day 7	Cranberry juice	½ cup

Give Your Brain a Daily Bath

Bathe your brain (the more times per day the better) in combinations of antioxidant/anti-inflammatory polyphenols and phytonutrients found in SuperFoods. Some of the most important polyphenols include anthocyanins/proanthocyanidins/ellagitannins, all of which can be found in berries and other fruits and veggies as well. Spinach, strawberry, and blueberry extracts have been shown to be effective in reversing age-related deficits in brain and behavior function in rats, with all three supplemental diets showing positive effects on cognitive behavior. Blueberries showed the greatest increases in motor performance and several measures of neuronal communication, demonstrating that it is really possible to increase the ability of old neurons to communicate with one another (yes, you can teach old neurons new tricks). A study published in 2006 in *Neurology* followed 3,718 people over the age of sixty-five. Those who ate at least 2.8 servings of vegetables a day (as compared to those who ate 1 or less) had a 40 percent slower rate of decline of cognitive ability. Spinach proved to be the most effective vegetable, which goes to prove that Popeye was not only strong; he was smart, too!

RESVERATROL AND YOUR GENES—AND GETTING YOUR BODY TO THINK IT'S EATING LESS

Recent studies have shown that resveratrol has potent antioxidant activity (which leads to decreased oxidative stress) and also has the ability to inhibit platelet aggregation (which means it decreases the risk of blood clot formation and therefore decreases risk of stroke and heart attack). These actions may help prevent free-radical damage throughout the body and provide protective support to the cardiovascular system. However, some of the most interesting studies have demonstrated that resveratrol turns on the genetic pathway in our body that mimics caloric restriction—a diet in which calorie intake is markedly reduced. Caloric restriction opposes the development of a broad spectrum of age-associated changes and, in all animal model tests to date, extends life span. It improves immune function and insulin sensitivity and reduces oxidative stress, all of which promote a health span that equals your life span. Most caloric restriction has been studied in animals, where the calories are restricted to around 60 to 70 percent of what the animal would normally eat, and a corresponding increase in life span of around 30 to 40 percent is seen. Caloric restriction, and potentially resveratrol, causes active alterations in the aging process by affecting anti-aging genes in the body. There have been no long-term studies in humans. This kind of caloric restriction is almost impossible to live by if you want to have enough energy to get through a busy day of working and taking care of a family. But the good news is that you may well get the biochemical benefits of caloric restriction by consuming resveratrol without actually being calorically restricted. I know I'd rather eat purple grapes than go on a strict low-calorie diet.

THE FUTURE OF NUTRIGENOMICS

The problem of designing a "nutrigenomics profile" that would map out the most ideal diet and lifestyle choices for every individual is, of course, multilayered. The human genome is estimated to encode more than 30,000 genes said to be responsible for generating more than 100,000 proteins. Understanding the interrelationships among genes, gene products, and dietary habits is fundamental to identifying those who will benefit most from or be placed at risk by intervention strategies. This understanding of complex traits and disorders in humans is further complicated by genetic variations between individuals, which, for example, may make one person become obese and develop diabetes, while another person, who makes what we would consider poor lifestyle choices, may not have a perceptible problem. Not to mention the fact that most chronic diseases are determined by a number of different genes and are caused by mechanisms that are difficult and complex. Therefore, the goal of a personalized diet for optimum health is not yet ready for prime time—but the recommendations in this book can certainly help us get there.

Here's my theory: Be kind to your genes. As much as possible, act like you're still a caveman or cavewoman. The human genome has changed less than 0.02 percent in the last forty thousand years. If you want to thrive as modern man or woman with Stone Age genes, you'd better try to do as much as possible to emulate the lifestyle and food choices that cavemen and cavewomen encountered. That means lots of whole foods (SuperFoods) found in nature and lots of outdoor activities.

We may not yet have all the answers. But it's important to recognize that these twenty-five Super-Foods and fifteen SuperNutrients and their sidekicks and lifestyle choices have positive health effects on our genomes and the expression of genetic information contained in them. For instance, there's never going to be a headline that says, "Sleep Is Bad for Your Health!" or "Blueberry: The Little Blue Devil That Kills!" I'm not asking you to step into dangerous territory. What I'd like is for all of us to get our lifestyle and food choices to line up with our genetic heritage.

Eventually health care will include the complete genetic profiling of every individual, assessing her or his risk for acquiring nutrition-related disorders. At the moment we have little idea of all the genetic factors and how they will interact. Until more is known, advice based on simple testing must remain simple as well—for example, drink less alcohol or eat less saturated fat. So that's what I tell you to do. But think about this: Since each of the SuperFoods and SuperNutrients and the six steps in this book have a positive influence, taken all together there must be any number of factors that will help to regulate your specific genome in a favorable way. For the complete Week 1 Daily Planner, see page 287.

◆ MEET SPIRO CHACONOS ◆

A Late Bloomer Catches Up

Spiro Chaconos was what some might call a natural athlete. He excelled at both football and baseball, went to Northwestern on an athletic scholarship, and was drafted by the Detroit Tigers right out of college. The problem was he got accepted to dental school at the same time.

"Here I was at the age of twenty," he says, "and making the biggest decision of my life." This was in the early sixties, when pro baseballers made about $6,000 a year. When Chaconos's uncle, a dentist with an established practice, told him how much more than $6,000 he made a year, the decision became a lot less difficult. And Chaconos became a dentist—an orthodontist, actually, and one of the most well respected in his field. He also taught at UCLA for twenty-six years. He kept his hand in athletics as the football team's dentist (he also did stints for the Philadelphia Eagles and the Kansas City Chiefs). As for his own athletics, he stayed active, mostly running five or six miles around the track—until his back went out, and he had to have surgery, which laid him up for six months.

"After that I used my back as an excuse not to exercise. I wasn't pushing myself away from the table very well, either. Like a lot of other athletes, I had been used to eating a lot and working it off. Well, I kept eating a lot, but I was no longer working it off. I was overeating, overdrinking, and overpartying."

Then, at the age of fifty-five, the self-described "late bloomer" got married and soon had two sons who are now ages ten and eleven. He also had high blood pressure and high cholesterol.

"I coach my sons' baseball teams," he says, "and I realized I wanted to be around for a long time to see them play. So about six months ago, I embarked on the SuperHealth program. I eat all the SuperFoods, from walnuts to blueberries, to loads of fruits and vegetables. I planted my own vegetable garden, so I've always got organic greens. I planted an avocado tree in my yard. I actually carry a deck of cards and a tennis ball around with me so I know what size portions I should be eating. I'm now working out again. I started at 225, and now I'm down to 191 and still going. My cholesterol and blood pressure readings are both down significantly. In fact, my doctor just took me off my medication."

The biggest difference for Spiro is in his energy level. "About a year ago," he says, "I couldn't make it through the day without wanting to take a nap. I was tired all the time, and I couldn't sleep at night. I was taking over-the-counter sleeping pills. Now I fall asleep the minute my head touches the pillow and I sleep a good seven hours straight. And I finally feel that I have a chance of living a long, healthy life."

Step 2:
Become an Environmentalist
and Detox Your Body

*For your basics, see the SuperHealth Food Pyramid,
page 19 (for your bonus, see below)*

Week 2 SuperFoods:

Soy	Garlic
Apples	Broccoli
Tea	Spices
Onions	

You are only as healthy as the environment in which you
live. If your internal environment is full of protective
warriors like omega-3 fatty acids, antioxidants, and phytonutrients, you are building a fort to keep toxic substances from getting into your body, and you are arming
yourself to fight off the ones that do. If your external environment—like your house—is not conducive to good
health (and it won't be if you use pesticides and many
traditional cleaning products), and that's where you lay
your head to sleep every night, you could be in a bit of
trouble—high blood pressure, heart disease, stroke, cancer, asthma, atopic skin disorders can all be influenced
by the environment. The same with your yard and your
surroundings. If you make it a place where the birds and

bees can thrive, it will be a place where you can thrive as well. By maintaining a healthy environment inside and out, you stand a much better chance of getting into the SuperHealth zone and staying there.

Keeping yourself in the SuperHealth "green" zone is not as difficult as it may seem. In this chapter you'll find:

- Foods to counteract internal and external toxins
- Steps to take to detoxify your home
- Ways to combat the effects of outdoor pollutants

Going green leads to a healthier environment, and a healthier environment leads to a healthier you. For instance, choosing the particular foods in this chapter can help block certain cancer cells from forming and growing. By using nontoxic, biodegradable products in our homes and offices, we can dramatically reduce the number of potentially cancer-causing agents to which we are exposed. By keeping your air conditioner in top working order, you can reduce the indoor air pollution that can worsen the symptoms and severity of respiratory diseases such as asthma and chronic obstructive pulmonary disease.

FIGHTING OFF TOXINS WITH FOODS

The best way to avoid the effects of toxins such as pesticides and industrial waste is to avoid foods that have these toxins in them or on them or those that may have been contaminated by them. One way to do that is to eat organic. Organic foods are grown without the use of conventional pesticides or chemical fertilizers and are processed without additives. If animal products are labeled ORGANIC, it means the animal was given organic feed, and not given substances like antibiotics and growth hormones. By eating organic we don't get the chemicals in our bodies that potentially could cause cancer, heart disease, and respiratory ailments.

However, it's really more important that you consume plenty of fruits and veggies than to worry about whether or not they're organic. First make sure you're including as many SuperFoods as possible in your diet. Then, if you can afford it, go organic. If you have a limited budget for organic foods, then use it for spinach and whole grains, because they are grown using more pesticides than other foods. I support organic farming whenever and wherever I can, but if I'm somewhere that organic food is not available, I don't stress about it. Better to build up your army of internal warriors—vitamins, minerals, phytonutrients, polyphenols—with the foods you are able to find and afford.

EATING GREEN

In step two of our SuperHealth Plan, we're adding seven foods and nutrients: soy, apples, tea, onions, cruciferous vegetables, garlic, and spices. These foods will help reduce the harmful effects of those toxins that do slip in.

Soy

Recommended amounts: 10 to 15 grams of soy protein daily (if you're a breast cancer survivor, talk to your oncologist about soy consumption). You have to check the labels of soy foods to discover how many grams of protein they contain, as different types and brands can vary greatly. However, here are some examples:

Edamame	1 cup (1 baseball)	23 grams
Tofu	4 ounces (1 deck of cards)	18–20 grams
Tempeh	½ cup (½ baseball)	16–19 grams
Soy nuts	¼ cup (1 layer on your palm)	15 grams
Soymilk	1 cup (8 ounces)	7–11 grams

The soybean is a legume with tremendous health benefits. It is a great and complete alternative protein.

Soy protein is now recognized as the only complete protein from a plant source, which means soy protein contains all of the essential amino acids that you must get from food, as the body cannot manufacture them. Soy protects against environmental toxins because it prevents certain cancer cells from forming and reproducing. It has also been shown to help reduce cholesterol, lower blood pressure, reduce the risk of cancer, and help relieve menstrual and menopausal symptoms. There is some controversy about soy and whether or not it raises the risk of breast cancer. However, I believe that soy is a safe and healthful food when eaten as a whole-food form (I am not in favor of isoflavone-enriched food or supplements, which use only one part of the soybean—for whole foods to give you all their nutrient value, they must remain whole).

Why is soy a good protector of your internal environment? The main reason is that soy, in all the forms listed in the next section, is loaded with phytoestrogens, plant-based chemicals that are weaker versions of the human hormone estrogen. They give you all the benefits of estrogen—for example, decreased risk for cardiovascular disease and osteoporosis—and none of the potential harmful side effects. One of the functions of estrogen is to bind to specific sites on cell membranes called estrogen receptors to promote the proliferation of cells in places like the breast and uterus. While this is a normal function of the body, it can get out of hand and stimulate the growth of tumors. Phytoestrogens also bind to these estrogen receptors. So if they get there first, they become warriors that block the more potent hormones from producing cancer cells. Many environmental toxins also have the ability to bind to estrogen receptors, and they, too, can be blocked by phytoestrogens. Soy is also a protease inhibitor, which means it plays a role in healthy cell regulation. It inhibits chemical carcinogens (for example, industrial pollutants) from becoming activated and keeps them from causing cells to become malignant.

Soy and Iodine

If you are a soy lover, it's important that you take a multivitamin that contains iodine. People who are iodine deficient can have thyroid dysfunction when they consume soy because it can cause thyroid hormone imbalances. This is especially important, as the SuperHealth program advocates staying away from salt, which is often iodized. So check the label of your multivitamin, and look for the ingredient "iodine."

Soy Sidekicks to Help Fight Damaging Toxins

- **Tofu** is made by coagulating soymilk, and then pressing the resulting curds into blocks. There are many different varieties of tofu, including firm, extra-firm, soft, and silken. Tofu has very little flavor or smell on its own, so it can be seasoned or marinated to suit the dish. Firm tofu can be baked, broiled, or grilled and is good used in stir-fries and soups. Silken tofu can be made into tasty smoothies, dips, and dressings. Tofu should be kept refrigerated in a covered, water-filled container. Change the water it soaks in daily and, since it's perishable, be sure to check the expiration date on the package.
- **Soymilk** is made from soybeans that have been ground, cooked, and strained, and is a good choice for people who are lactose intolerant. You can sometimes find it fresh in the refrigerated dairy section of the supermarket, but now it most often comes in drink-box-type packaging, which means it will keep for a long time and does not have to be refrigerated until opened. Soymilk comes in many brands and flavors, so try several different ones until you find one you like. I use a cup in my cereal every morning; you can also use it in making smoothies, pancakes, muffins, and cakes. Just substitute it for milk in nearly any recipe. My two

favorite brands are Kirkland (from Costco) and Silk.

- **Soy yogurt** is made by fermenting soymilk with friendly bacteria, and it contains natural probiotics. The process is similar to the production of yogurt from cow's milk. It comes in a variety of flavors, just like dairy yogurt. It is not as easy to find in the supermarket as soymilk, but is usually available in health food stores and chains like Whole Foods and Trader Joe's.

- **Soy nuts** are soybeans that have been soaked in water and then baked or roasted until they're lightly browned. They're high in protein, phytoestrogens, and fiber—but they're also high in calories, so I recommend no more than ¼ cup per day (one layer on your palm). When buying, read the label to make sure there is no added salt, oil, or sweetener. Soy nuts are good anytime as a snack, or the way I like them—tossed on top of my morning cereal.

- **Edamame** are green soybeans still in their pods. Edamame can be eaten as a snack or a vegetable dish, or used in soups, stews, pasta, or salads. For a snack, lightly boil the pods in salted water, then squeeze the seeds directly from the pods into your mouth with your fingers. You can also buy frozen edamame, which makes it even easier to prepare.

- **Tempeh** is a cake of soybeans that have been dehulled, cooked, and mixed with grains and other flavorings. It can be found in the refrigerated section of your health food store or supermarket. It has a somewhat nutty flavor, and it is often used as a meat substitute in cooking. It can be marinated and grilled or added to chili, pasta sauces, sloppy joes, or burritos.

- **Miso** is made from fermented soybeans and sometimes a grain such as rice or wheat combined with salt and a friendly mold culture, and then aged in cedar vats for one to three years. In the United States it is best known in the form of miso soup, but it can also be used as a condiment. It is, however, high in sodium, so is best used sparingly. It is usually available in health food stores either packed in sealed plastic bags or in glass jars. After opening, a package of miso will keep for several months in the fridge.

Apples

Recommended amounts: 1 apple daily (1 baseball)
Sidekick: pears

When Mom said, "An apple a day . . . ," she knew what she was talking about. A number of studies have shown that apple consumption protects pulmonary function (which is often compromised by poor air quality) and is associated with reduced risk for a number of diseases, including cancer—particularly lung cancer—as well as asthma, cardiovascular disease, and type 2 diabetes.

Apples contain high levels of an antioxidant flavonoid called quercetin (which is also found abundantly in onions, tea, and red wine) and may be important in protecting the lungs from the harmful effects of atmospheric pollutants and cigarette smoke. A 2007 study found that children who drank apple juice at least once a day were half as likely to suffer from wheezing, often a sign of asthma, as those drinking it less than once a month. Researchers believe that the phytochemicals in apples help to calm the inflammation in the airways, which is a key feature of both wheezing and asthma.

Apples are also filled with superantioxidants. The antioxidant activity of approximately one apple is equivalent to about 1500 milligrams of vitamin C, even though the amount of vitamin C in one apple is only about 5.7 milligrams. And where is most of that antioxidant activity found? In the apple peel. In fact, the peel is anywhere from two to six times more antioxidant rich than the flesh of the apple. So when you eat an apple, eat it peel and all. And choose a wide variety of apples. Different varieties have different skin colors, meaning the phytonutrient content of the skin varies in concentration and type. In the United States, Fuji and Red Delicious apples have the highest polyphenol and flavonoid (antioxidant, anti-inflammatory warriors) content, but variety is still key.

Tea

Recommended amounts: 4 or more 8-ounce cups daily

Tea is hot these days. And it's cold. Everywhere you go, tea is being served and sold in previously unimaginable flavor blends. That's because tea is not only a delicious brew; it's full of health benefits that can be yours for very little effort and very little cost. Tea is an anti-inflammatory that helps decrease the cancer-promoting properties of environmental toxins, and it can help decrease body fat, which is where our bodies store many environmental toxins. Regular tea consumption has also been shown to help lower blood pressure, prevent cardiovascular disease, strengthen bones and gums, protect against skin cancer, decrease sun-induced aging of the skin, and boost your metabolism.

There are four types of tea: white, green, black, and oolong. They all come from the same *Camellia sinensis* plant; the difference comes from how the tea leaves are processed. It used to be thought that green tea was the healthiest to drink, but recent studies have shown that each of the four teas has different phytonutrient profiles, all of which provide health benefits. Processing may make a slight difference in the amount of flavonoids, but not enough to make a significant difference in how they affect your health, and particularly during this week of environmental detox. Most of the health studies have been done on green tea, but it's probably a good idea to mix up your tea choices, as the sum of all the different nutrient profiles is better than any one by itself. Green is my tea of choice, simply because I like it best, but I do have a few cups of black tea a week as well. All you need to do is find a tea you like to drink and indulge. And don't forget, tea has no calories.

Tea is rich in flavonoids. In 2003 Harvard scientists found that tea acts as a sort of natural vaccine that "teaches" immune cells to recognize markers on the surface of invading toxins. When participants drank five or six cups of tea a day, there was an increased production of an important disease-fighting protein on their immune system T cells. This means that in a toxic environment, tea helps us to fight off foreign invaders that could potentially lead to ailments like cancer and cardiovascular disease.

The healthful compounds in tea also help prevent the formation of new blood vessels that usually accompanies the growth of malignant tissue. Tumor cells release chemicals to encourage blood vessel growth so that they will be fed and can grow. Drinking tea helps to inhibit that process. By the way, black pepper and citrus help increase the body's ability to absorb the bioactive "goodies" in tea. So if you add pepper to your lunch or dinner, have a cup of tea afterward to get the most benefits. Or if you have a cup of tea, take one or two swallows of orange juice or eat an orange section right before or after.

Concerned About Caffeine?

Tea does contain caffeine, but much less than you'll find in a cup of coffee. White tea has about 90 percent less caffeine than coffee, while black tea has about 50 percent less caffeine. The good news is that many types of tea now come in decaffeinated versions. And if you're using loose-leaf tea and brewing it, you can decaffeinate it yourself. Here's how: Brew a pot or cup of tea, then drain out the liquid. Most of the caffeine goes down the spout with the tea! Then pour some more hot water over your leaves and you have a cup or pot of decaf tea. Simple.

It is important to note that the term "herbal tea" traditionally refers to infusions of fruits or herbs and typically contains no actual tea. The herbal tea I most often recommend is rooibos, or South African red tea, which is naturally caffeine free and contains a wide array of phytonutrients. It is one of the only herbal teas with a significant body of scientific literature to support the health claims associated with its consumption (it is anticarcinogenic, anti-inflammatory, and antiviral). Two brands I enjoy are Numi (www.numitea.com) and Tetley's Rooibos Vanilla Pear Herbal Tea (www.tetleyusa.com).

ORGANOSULFUR COMPOUNDS AND THE BEST SOURCES OF ORGANOSULFUR COMPOUNDS

Organosulfurs are important because they help "turn on" one of the body's first lines of defense against cancer: Phase 2 detoxification enzymes (nutrigenomics at its best; this is a prime example of a food turning on a beneficial genetic pathway in our body). These enzymes are central to the body's ability to protect itself from all manner of carcinogens (such as pesticides and industrial waste) that routinely enter our bodies through the food we eat, the water we drink, the air we breathe, and our skin. When they are activated, Phase 2 enzymes can go on the attack against carcinogens and render them inert so that they can be excreted from the body.

What do onions, broccoli, and tea have in common? They are all full of flavonoids. Onions (and their sidekicks on page 55) contain generous amounts of quercetin, which has been shown to protect against cataracts, cardiovascular disease, and cancer. Studies have shown that quercetin and other flavonoids have the ability to modify the human body's reaction to allergens, viruses, and carcinogens. After we eat foods that are rich in flavonoids like quercetin, antioxidant activity in the bloodstream increases, enzymes that help eliminate mutagens and carcinogens are released, and mechanisms that help kill cancer cells are induced.

In addition, organosulfur compounds have been linked to lowering blood pressure and cholesterol levels and helping to prevent heart disease and cancer. Cruciferous vegetables like broccoli and its sidekicks (see the list on page 55) are also potent organosulfurs.

Chew Your Way to Better Health

If you want to get the most out of your organosulfurs (and I know you do), then chop them up and let them sit for about ten minutes before you cook them or eat them in order to activate their nutrients and anticancer chemical compounds. Cutting, cooking, and freezing can all activate the nutrients. If you're eating these veggies raw, chew them for at least fifteen seconds so that the fibers get broken up, which begins the activation process. Alternate between eating the veggies raw and cooked. The best way to cook them is to lightly steam them in stainless steel cookware or microwave them in a little bit of water. Stir-frying also preserves most of the anticancer chemicals in cruciferous vegetables.

In the best of all possible worlds, you'd grow your vegetables in your yard and eat them within hours of picking. Fresh vegetables bought in the store may not be as fresh as we'd like because they probably were picked several days earlier and shipped to your store. Frozen vegetables, however, are often better than fresh, because they're usually frozen shortly after they're picked. In the end, however, it comes down to this: There is no bad way to eat a vegetable.

Onions

Recommended amount: ⅛ to ¼ medium onion (⅛ to ¼ baseball) or sidekick most days
Sidekicks: scallions, shallots, leeks, chives, garlic

Garlic

Recommended amount: to taste, as often as you like, at least daily
Sidekicks: scallions, shallots, leeks, chives, onion

Broccoli

Recommended amount: 1 cup (1 baseball) daily
Sidekicks: broccoli sprouts, Brussels sprouts, red and green cabbage, kale, turnips, cauliflower, collards, bok choy, mustard greens, Swiss chard, rutabaga, kohlrabi, broccoflower, arugula, watercress, daikon root, wasabi, liverwort

One of the anticancer chemicals in broccoli, indole-3-carbinol, acts like a phytoestrogen, just like soy. It helps reduce the effects of pollutants like dioxin that can affect your hormones (dioxin gets into our systems through fat from food—the reason you should trim the fat and skin off any meat you're going to eat is that that's where all the toxins are stored); indole-3-carbinol and phytoestrogens block these harmful substances from binding with estrogen receptors.

Absolute musts: If there's only one organosulfur food you add daily for this week, or if you're traveling and can't control your diet, my recommendation is broccoli sprouts.

Had Your Broccoli Sprouts Lately?

Broccoli sprouts are the most potent source of organosulfurs, containing extremely high concentrations of a helpful phytonutrient called sulforaphane. In fact, concentrations of sulforaphane and other cancer-fighting substances are from twenty to fifty times higher in three-day-old broccoli sprouts than in mature plants. Broccoli sprouts, which look and taste very much like alfalfa sprouts, can be found in many supermarket chains like Wal-Mart and ShopRite, but if you can't locate them in your area, you can find them on the Internet at www.broccosprouts.com. They can be used in salads or as sandwich fillings, as in this recipe for a turkey baguette: Take one French baguette, cut it into two 6-inch lengths, and then slice it lengthwise. Spread on mustard to taste. Place salad greens, 1 sliced tomato, 1 sliced onion, and ¼ pound sliced turkey on the bread. Top with 1 cup of broccoli sprouts. This makes 2 servings.

Spices

Recommended amounts: As much as you like, to taste, as often as you like

If you're like most people in the United States, you probably use spices to boost the flavors of your favorite dishes. What you may not realize is that when you cook with spices, you're boosting your health as well. All spices, which are derived from tree bark, seeds, or fruit, help to detoxify the body. They are part of your environmental shield, as they rev up Phase 2 enzymes that block cancer, and they help further reduce cancer risk by stimulating apoptosis, or programmed cell death. Your body has the ability to identify unhealthy cells; it first tries to help sick cells, and if they don't respond, it sends them a "death star" and kills them off. When programmed cell death does not work right, cells that should be eliminated may hang around and become immortal; for example, in cancer and leukemia.

The Best Spices

All spices have health benefits. They are all potent anti-inflammatories. However, one of the most potent SuperHealth spices is turmeric, because it contains curcumin, which gives it its yellow-orange color. A natural detoxifier, curcumin helps protect the liver from the damaging effects of alcohol, toxic chemicals, and even some pharmaceutical drugs. Laboratory research has shown curcumin to be a potent anti-inflammatory associated with providing relief for rheumatoid arthritis, as well as helping to prevent heart disease and cancer. Studies show that curcumin may also help to prevent Alzheimer's disease.

I especially recommend:

- Anise for its anti-inflammatory properties and because it promotes pulmonary health
- Black pepper because it enhances the absorption of polyphenols and has antioxidant and anticancer properties
- Caraway because it promotes digestive health and has antimicrobial action
- Cayenne because it promotes cardiovascular and gastrointestinal health and pain relief and enhances immunity
- Cinnamon for its healthful effects on blood sugar and cholesterol levels
- Clove for its anticancer, anti-inflammatory properties
- Coriander because it promotes healthy lipid (fat) profiles and has antidiabetic properties
- Cumin for its detoxification properties
- Fennel because it promotes digestive health
- Fenugreek for its antidiabetic properties

- Ginger for its antioxidant, anticancer, anti-inflammatory properties
- Licorice for its anti-inflammatory, antibacterial, anticancer, and phytoestrogen properties
- Marjoram because it helps atopic skin diseases and is possibly protective against Alzheimer's disease
- Nutmeg for its anti-inflammatory and anticancer properties
- Oregano for its antioxidant, antifungal, antibacterial, and lung protection properties
- Rosemary for its antioxidant, anti-inflammatory, detoxification properties
- Saffron for its anticancer properties
- Sage for its antioxidant properties
- Thyme for its anticancer properties
- Turmeric for its cancer-fighting and Alzheimer's disease prevention properties

Absolute musts: Curcumin is available in supplement form. If there's only one spice you add for the week, or if you're traveling and can't control your diet, my recommendation is to take two 500-milligram capsules a day, or take the SuperFoodsRx Spice Supplement.

My Favorite Spicy Soda

If you're looking for a fun way to add spice to your life, try my favorite spicy soda, Virgil's Root Beer (www.virgils.com). It's made from anise, licorice, vanilla, cinnamon, cloves, wintergreen, sweet birch, molasses, nutmeg, pimento berry oil, balsam oil, and oil of cassia.

Week 2: Green Eating Daily Planner

The chart below is an example of how you can add environmentally friendly foods to your SuperHealth program, but it doesn't mean these are the only foods you should eat for the week. These are just suggestions; feel free to mix and match foods and days to your heart's content (and health).

	Food Suggestion	**Daily Servings**
Day 1	Soy nuts	¼ cup (1 layer on your palm)
	Apple	1 medium (1 baseball)
	Broccoli sprouts	2 cups (2 baseballs)
	Onion	¼ medium (¼ baseball)
	Garlic	To taste
	Spices	To taste
	Tea	4 cups (32 ounces)
Day 2	Tofu	½ cup raw tofu (½ baseball)
	Apple	1 medium (1 baseball)
	Brussels sprouts (raw or cooked)	2 cups (2 baseballs, raw or cooked)
	Chives	¼ cup (¼ baseball)
	Garlic	To taste
	Spices	To taste
	Tea	4 cups (32 ounces)
Day 3	Edamame	1 cup (1 baseball)
	Pear	1 medium (1 baseball)
	Red cabbage (raw or cooked)	1–2 cups (1–2 baseballs) raw, ½ cup cooked (½ baseball)
	Leeks (raw or cooked)	¼ cup (¼ baseball) raw or cooked
	Garlic	To taste
	Spices	To taste
	Tea	4 cups (32 ounces)
Day 4	Soy yogurt	One 6-ounce container
	Apple	1 medium (1 baseball)
	Kale (raw or cooked)	2 cups (2 baseballs) raw, ½ cup cooked (½ baseball)
	Onion	¼ medium (¼ baseball)
	Garlic	To taste
	Spices	To taste
	Tea	4 cups (32 ounces)
Day 5	Soymilk	2 cups (16 ounces)
	Apple	1 medium (1 baseball)

(continued)

	Food Suggestion	Daily Servings
Day 5 (cont.)	Broccoli (raw or cooked)	2 cups (2 baseballs) raw or cooked
	Chives	¼ medium (¼ baseball)
	Garlic	To taste
	Spices	To taste
	Tea	4 cups (32 ounces)
Day 6	Tempeh	½ cup (½ baseball)
	Pear	1 medium (1 baseball)
	Collard greens (raw or cooked)	2 cups (2 baseballs) raw, ½ cup cooked (½ baseball)
	Scallions	¼ cup (¼ baseball)
	Garlic	To taste
	Spices	To taste
	Tea	4 cups (32 ounces)
Day 7	Tofu	½ cup raw tofu (½ baseball)
	Apple	1 medium (1 baseball)
	Broccoli sprouts	2 cups (2 baseballs)
	Onion	¼ medium (¼ baseball)
	Garlic	To taste
	Spices	To taste
	Tea	4 cups (32 ounces)

Mom's Citrus Suggestion

When I was growing up, my mother made sure we had our citrus fruit for vitamin C. But, unlike most other moms, she also insisted that we eat a few bites of the skin and all the white membrane beneath (the part that most kids hate). I still do it today. It doesn't taste great, but it turns out that citrus skin contains monoterpenoids, compounds that inhibit carcinogen activation (carcinogens have to be activated in your body to cause a problem). If you can't swallow the idea of eating citrus skins, try making a recipe or two that include citrus zest (see page 281). Or use Kirkland's Organic No Salt Seasoning, which contains orange and lemon peel (I put it on just about everything I eat).

ADDITIONAL DETOXIFIERS

Because we live in the real world, there is no way we can avoid every toxin there is. If we tried, we might miss out on some important health benefits. Take fish, for instance. We know from the Control Your Genes chapter that the omega-3s found in many fish help turn on good genes that can keep us moving toward SuperHealth. Fish and shellfish contain high-quality protein and other essential nutrients, are low in saturated fat, and contain omega-3 fatty acids. A well-balanced diet that includes a variety of fish and shellfish can contribute to heart health and children's proper growth and development. So women of childbearing age and young children in particular should include fish or shellfish in their diets for their many nutritional benefits.

However, nearly all fish and shellfish contain traces of mercury. Mercury is a heavy metal that occurs naturally in the environment and can also be released into the air through industrial pollution. There is mercury used in dental fillings as well. While some experts are concerned that the release of microscopic amounts of mercury into the body may cause kidney or neurological damage, others, including the American Dental Association, say that these minute amounts of mercury cause no damage. Mercury can accumulate in streams and oceans and is turned into methylmercury in the water, which is then consumed by the fish in those waters. It is this type of mercury that can be harmful to an unborn baby and young child, causing effects such as mental retardation, seizures, cerebral palsy, abnormal gait and/or speech, and problems in vision and hearing. This is why women of reproductive age need to be especially careful about their fish intake.

Here's what you can do to make sure you're consuming minimal levels of mercury:

- **Choose fish and shellfish that are lower in mercury.** Five of the most commonly eaten types of seafood that are low in mercury are shrimp, canned light tuna, wild salmon, farmed tilapia, and farmed catfish. Another commonly eaten fish, albacore ("white") tuna, has more mercury than canned light tuna. So, when choosing your two to four meals per week of fish and shellfish, you should eat no more than 6 ounces of albacore tuna per week. I eat wild salmon four to five times a week. Any trace amounts of mercury that might be in the fish are so small as to be harmless. The same goes for sardines, as they are small fish that aren't around long enough to pick up enough harmful toxins to make a big difference.

Add a Little Yogurt

Here's a little-known fact: The active cultures in yogurt change the mercury in fish to a less toxic form. So you don't have to go out and buy mercury-laden fish and cook it in yogurt—but if you're going to have fish, a ½-cup serving of yogurt for dessert will help detoxify any mercury that's lurking around.

- **Get more selenium in your diet.** Selenium is a good protector against mercury toxicity. It also helps rev up glutathione, the body's primary intracellular protector, which in turn decreases oxidative stress that could be caused by the mercury, and oxidation is a precursor to all disease (heart disease, cancer, diabetes, and so on). Aim for 70 to 100 micrograms of selenium a day from a combination of the following foods:
  - 3 ounces cooked Pacific oysters = 131 mcg
  - 1 cup whole wheat flour = 85 mcg
  - ⅓ can Pacific sardines (about 2 ounces) = 75 mcg
  - 1 dried Brazil nut = 68 to 91 mcg
  - 3 ounces canned white tuna = 56 mcg
  - 3 ounces cooked clams = 54 mcg
  - 6 farmed oysters = 54 mcg

- 3 ounces roasted skinless turkey breast = 27 mcg
- ¼ cup sunflower seeds = 21 mcg
- 1 cup brown rice = 19 mcg

Selenium can also be taken in a multivitamin (such as the SuperFoodsRx multivitamin).

- **Monitor your sushi consumption.** In January 2008 *The New York Times* conducted a test of tuna sushi from a number of high-end New York restaurants. They found that six pieces of tuna sushi from most of the eateries contained more than 49 micrograms of mercury—the amount that the EPA deems acceptable for weekly consumption over a period of several months. These findings reinforce results in other studies showing that more expensive tuna usually contains more mercury because it is more likely to come from a larger species, which accumulates mercury from the fish it eats. But there's no need to panic. According to the Food and Drug Administration, one week's consumption doesn't change the level of methylmercury in the body much at all. But be sure to monitor the mercury level of the fish consumed. My advice? Beware of excessive consumption of tuna sushi—once a month is probably fine.
- **Do not eat shark, swordfish, king mackerel, or tilefish** because they contain high levels of mercury.

Mercury Updates

To get the latest updates on fish that are high in mercury or other toxins, or that have been overfished, visit the Monterey Bay Aquarium's Web site, www.mbayaq.org, and click on Seafood Watch. Other good sources are the Environmental Protection Agency (www.epa.gov/mercury/fish.htm), the Environmental Defense Fund (www.edf.org), and the Marine Stewardship Council (www.msc.org).

There are other pollutants, including lead, cadmium, and dioxins, that you can combat via healthful eating:

- **Get the lead out. Be sure your diet, and especially your children's diets, contains plenty of Super-Foods rich in iron and calcium.** Back in the 1970s and before, when we were either innocent or oblivious, depending on your point of view, houses were built with materials such as lead paint that were dangerous to your health and the health of your children. Lead is the most common carcinogenic metal in the environment, which is why lead is so dangerous. Problems arise when young children swallow paint particles, or when lead-based paint is improperly removed by dry scraping, sanding, or open-flame burning. You can also breathe in lead dust if you are renovating and disturb painted surfaces. Children who consume a healthy amount of iron and calcium absorb less lead. All iron is more bioavailable when you have vitamin C in the meal. Foods rich in iron include spinach, shiitake mushrooms, kidney beans, sesame seeds, pumpkin seeds, lentils, Swiss chard, tofu, green beans, kale, shrimp, broccoli, Brussels sprouts, soybeans, wheat germ, lima beans, green peas, skinless turkey breast, and lean red meat. Foods rich in calcium include collard greens, Swiss chard, kale, nonfat organic dairy products, low-fat cheese, fortified soymilk, broccoli, tofu, canned sardines and wild salmon (with bones), green beans, green peas, and almonds. Any vitamin C–containing foods (oranges, lemons, kiwis, pink grapefruits, tomatoes, broccoli, red, orange, yellow, and green peppers) or vitamin C supplement will enhance the absorption of iron.
- **Favoring calcium-rich foods also helps combat cadmium toxicity.** You can ingest cadmium if you eat plants grown in contaminated soil or fish that come from contaminated water, or if you drink contaminated water itself (which typically results from improper disposal of industrial chemicals).

Cadmium is also found in smoke from cigarettes. Cadmium toxicity can lead to hypertension, kidney dysfunction, glucose intolerance, dyslipidemia (high blood fat levels), and zinc deficiency. You probably would never know if you were ingesting too much cadmium, so the safest route is to include calcium in your diet as a preventive measure—so think nonfat milk (preferably organic, 1 to 2 cups a day), nonfat yogurt (preferably organic, 1 to 2 cups a day), and calcium-fortified soymilk (1 to 2 cups a day), as well as collard greens, Swiss chard, kale, low-fat cheese, broccoli, tofu, canned sardines and wild salmon (with bones), green beans, green peas, and almonds.

- **Un-saturate your diet to reduce dioxin exposure.** The best way to reduce your exposure to environmental dioxins is to reduce your intake, which means reducing your consumption of animal (saturated) fats. Dioxins are chemical compounds produced as by-products of combustion processes such as commercial or municipal waste incineration, copper smelting, chlorine pulp and paper bleaching, and from burning fuels (like wood, coal, or oil). The most common health effects of dioxin exposure include infertility, reduced sperm count, hormonal changes, endometriosis, and ovarian dysfunction. Several studies have also suggested that workers in the industries above who are exposed to high levels of dioxins over many years have an increased risk of cancer.

  Choose foods including:

  - Butter substitutes (for example, Smart Balance Lightly Salted Low Sodium Whipped Buttery Spread)
  - Wild Alaskan salmon
  - Skinless turkey breast
  - Buffalo (if it's not available in your area, you can get it online at Jackson Hole Buffalo Company [www.jhbuffalomeat.com] and Buffalo Gal

[www.buffalogal.com])
- Free-range grass-fed lean meat (found at stores like Whole Foods and Trader Joe's—my favorite brand is Niman Ranch [www.nimanranch.com])

Trim the excess fat from meat and choose the leanest cuts, such as top round, eye of round, or sirloin, and have no more than 3 to 4 ounces (1 deck of cards) a week. Stay away from foods that contain the highest concentration of dioxins, like high-fat cuts of beef, bacon, frankfurters, full-fat cheeses, butter, and fatty fish (such as farm-raised salmon).

A diet low in animal fats should start in childhood. Researchers have demonstrated an association between increasing half-life of dioxins and increasing age and adiposity—which means that the older you are and the heavier you are, the longer dioxins stay in your body— suggesting that the youngest children may be able to excrete these substances more readily. By adolescence the stability of these substances within the body becomes prolonged. So you can help your children live to be one hundred by instituting a diet that is relatively low in animal fat at a young age.

LIVING IN A HEALTHY HOUSE

When I was young my mother never had to tell us kids to go outside and play. That was what we did to have fun. Times and technology have changed the world, and because we now lead such sedentary lives, many of us spend as much as 90 percent of our time indoors. That's why it's so important that we do everything possible to make our homes and places of work as healthy and pollutant-free as possible.

"Greening up" your indoor environment has many health benefits, both short and long term, including helping to reduce or avoid both acute and chronic conditions such as:

Acute	**Chronic**
• Eye irritation/watering	• Cancer
• Nose irritation	• Liver damage
• Throat irritation	• Kidney damage
• Headaches	• Central nervous system
• Nausea/vomiting	damage
• Dizziness	• Endocrine (hormone)
• Asthma	imbalances

These conditions can be caused by what are known as volatile organic compounds, or VOCs, that are found in such everyday items as building materials, paints, furniture, cleaning products, automotive products, clothing, and even cosmetics. These products emit gases that we subsequently inhale.

Many state and local governments are beginning to take steps to reduce prospective pollutants in new homes. My hat is off to my home state of California for developing nonbinding guidelines (hey, it's a start) for the reduction of exposure to VOCs from construction materials in newly constructed or remodeled office buildings; other states have similar initiatives.

Every one of us can help improve our own health and the health of the planet by making our homes and offices "greener." Here are several simple steps you can take to give your home or office a detoxifying makeover:

- **Look for cleaning products that are nontoxic and biodegradable.** Read the label for these words. The word "organic" on the label doesn't tell you anything—right now the government has standards only for organic foods, so "organic" on a cleaning product can mean anything or nothing. Choose products with plant- and oil-based ingredients like grain alcohol, coconut oil, and eucalyptus instead of toxic chemicals like butyl cellosolve, petroleum, and triclosan. Cleaning ingredients vary in the type of health hazard they pose. Some cause acute, or immediate, hazards such as skin or respiratory irritation, watery eyes, or chemical burns, while others are associated with chronic or long-term effects such as cancer.

You can find nontoxic, biodegradable products in many supermarkets, health food stores, home improvement stores, and on the Internet. Here are a few suggested brands:

Seventh Generation (www.seventhgen.com)
Earth Friendly (www.ecos.com)
Simple Green (www.simplegreen.com)
Mrs. Meyers (www.mrsmeyers.com)
Ecover (www.ecover.com)
Dr. Bronner (www.drbronner.com)
Bio-Kleen (www.biokleen.com)

- **Make your own household cleaning products.** Ask your mother or your grandmother for their recipes—I know my mom had some great ones. You can find lots of them on the Internet, especially at sites like the Green Guide (www.thegreenguide.com); Arm & Hammer Baking Soda (www.armhammer.com); and the Vinegar Institute (www.versatilevinegar.org).

  Here are some of my favorite recipes:

  - *Fabric softener*: Add ¼ cup of baking soda to the wash cycle. Or add ¼ cup of white vinegar, as this will not only soften clothes; it will also eliminate static cling.
  - *Glass cleaner*: All you need to do is add ¼ cup of distilled vinegar to a 16-ounce spray bottle of warm water. Spray on glass and wipe with a soft cloth.
  - *Tub and tile cleaner*: Mix ¼ cup of borax (a naturally occurring mineral composed of sodium, boron, oxygen, and water, usually found in the cleaning aisle of your grocery store next to the powdered laundry soaps; the most common

brand is 20 Mule Team Borax) and ¼ cup of baking soda. Add 1½ cups of hot water and stir until mixed. Apply, scrub, and rinse.

- *All-purpose cleanser*: Mix equal parts water and white vinegar. Just wipe down the surface you want cleaned and let dry. You don't even have to rinse!
- *Drain cleaner*: Commercial drain cleaners can be highly toxic. Instead, pour ½ cup of baking soda down the drain, followed by ½ cup of white vinegar with a pinch of salt added. Rinse with hot water. Do this on a weekly basis and you'll prevent those nasty clogs.

- **Keep ventilation in mind: Open windows in your home and office whenever possible.** We can't totally avoid pollutants in our homes and offices. But we can minimize their harmful effects simply by opening windows, letting stale air out and fresh air in. Sleep with windows open at night (they don't have to be wide open—a small opening can help; you can use screens to keep bugs out). **Open your car windows** for a few minutes before you drive away. When the air in the car is heated by the sun, everything in it (the upholstery, the floor, the plastic cup holders) is emitting unhealthy VOCs. Opening the window lets those VOCs out so you can breathe easier when you get in. **Keep your kitchen properly ventilated.** Every time you cook, your house is polluted with smoke, soot, and carbon monoxide. If you have a gas stove, check your burners: If the flames are yellow-tipped, your stove may be releasing too much carbon monoxide (in which case, you should call the manufacturer and find out if the burners can be readjusted).
- **Keep your air conditioner in tip-top condition.** These blowers are great for helping to filter out many allergens. But if the filter is dirty, the AC may actually be distributing allergens throughout the room or house. Be sure to clean or replace the fil-

ter regularly. (Since there are so many different brands and types, read your manual or call the manufacturer to find out how often filters need to be cleaned.)

- **Conduct an energy audit of your house.** One-fifth of the entire energy consumption in the United States is in the home. Call your local utility company and they can either do an audit for you or tell you how you can get one done. An audit will check for leaks, evaluate your insulation levels, inspect heating and cooling equipment, and ensure you are using energy-efficient appliances and lightbulbs. If you fix all your leaky windows, replace your old stove, and improve inefficient heating and cooling, it not only will save you several hundred dollars a year; it will positively affect your health by decreasing the pollutants inside your house. You can clean up your environment while cleaning up the excess use of energy in your home.

Good Neighbors

Small actions at home can make a big difference in the fight against pollution. The National Wildlife Federation recently created the Good Neighbor Pledge, which asks signers to complete a checklist of environmentally friendly changes they will make around the house, such as installing compact fluorescent lightbulbs, buying energy-efficient appliances, and planting native trees. I urge you all to visit www.nwf.org/goodneighbor and take the pledge.

Be aware, however, that there is some controversy over fluorescent lightbulbs, because they contain mercury, and no one knows how to dispose of them. It looks like the best technology for the future, from an environmental standpoint, will be using be using solar-powered LED (light-emitting diode) lights.

- **Keep your house green.** One of the easiest ways to detoxify your home is to add houseplants. Many plants absorb chemicals that are harmful to humans and either convert them into food or destroy them by their own biological processes. Either way they thrive, and so do we! Ideally you should have at least two or three plants per 100 square feet of space. Keep plants near your computer as well as in your bedroom and living room. According to *Organic Gardening*, the top air-cleaning plants are:
  - Areca palm
  - Reed palm
  - Dwarf date palm
  - Boston fern
  - Pothos
  - English ivy
  - Australian sword fern
  - Peace lily
  - Rubber plant
  - Weeping fig
  - Dracaena

  Two or three houseplants will make a big difference for the average room and may reduce air toxicity levels by 75 percent. Put plants close to where you sit, work, and sleep rather than across the room.

- **Go green without going crazy.** There are so many simple things you can do to live in a "greener" world:
  - *Take your own fabric shopping bag to the grocery store* so you don't have to use their paper or plastic bags.
  - *Cook at home one additional night a week.* It saves a drive to a restaurant and take-out container waste.
  - *Eat one vegetarian meal a week.* Animal protein production uses more resources than vegetable protein production.

- *Cut shower time by two minutes.* You'll save water and energy.
- *Turn your cell phone off every once in a while.* So far no studies have shown a definitive link between cell phones and brain cancer, but because it's a new technology, we're not yet sure of long-term effects. There have been a few studies, however, that seem to indicate we should be cautious about cell phone use: A 2008 meta-analysis evaluated the EMF (electromagnetic field exposure) emitted by GSM (Global System for Mobile) phones and concluded that EMF exposure may have a small negative impact on memory and attention (by decreasing reaction time). An Israeli study concluded that regular or heavy users of cell phones showed "consistently elevated risks for parotid gland [the major salivary gland for the mouth] tumors." It's also been reported that cell phone use may alter protein expression in certain human cells, such as the endothelial cells that line the blood vessels and skin cells, although the significance of these alterations is not yet known and will require further studies. And, finally, a study that looked at semen quality in men attending an infertility clinic found that the use of cell phones decreased semen quality in men "by decreasing the sperm count motility, viability, and normal morphology." The degree of decrease was dependent on the duration of daily exposure to cell phones. It is clear that this is an ongoing area of research, and that with the passage of time and continued cell phone use, there is the possibility of potential harm to humans—especially children—and that limiting our exposure in a rational, nonalarmist fashion now hopefully will diminish our chances of developing adverse events from long-term extensive cell phone usage. So when using your cell phone, switch from one ear to the other weekly, limit the use of cell phones for children and adolescents, use headphones (and not always Bluetooth), and use your cell on speakerphone whenever you can.

- *Do some errands on foot.* You'll save gas, oil, antifreeze, brake fluid, and so on.
- *Get a copy of* National Geographic's quarterly *Green Guide*, a print and online magazine dedicated to showing consumers ways to gradually and affordably go green (www.thegreenguide.com). They also offer a free weekly e-newsletter.
- *Drive a little slower.* Don't be in such a hurry to get where you're going. Enjoy the ride. You'll burn less gas getting there.

For More Information . . .

If you want to be more environmentally responsible in your home and office, here are some resources you might want to check out: *Home Safe Home: Protecting Yourself and Your Family from Everyday Toxins and Harmful Household Products* by Debra Lynn Dadd (Tarcher/Penguin); the program Healthy Indoor Air for America's Homes (www.healthy indoorair.org); the Environmental Health Network (415-541-5075, www.ehnca.org); and the Consumer Product Safety Commission (800-638-CPSC, www.cpsc.gov). If you're building a new home, contact the National Association of Home Builders to find out how to get a "green" certification for your house (800-368-5242, www.nahb.org).

LIVING IN A HEALTHY WORLD

When I was growing up my mother refused to use pesticides or herbicides. She just allowed whatever grew in the grass to be part of the lawn. Her theory was to just water the lawn and mow it frequently (which was my job—and the only "power" we had in our mower came from my skinny legs) and it would remain green and healthy. And she was right, as always. She used no fertilizer, either; anything in her lawn had to be hardy enough to look good as it was.

I'm not saying that everything we grow should be

done without help or damage control. The U.S. Department of Agriculture reminds us that without pesticides many native habitats would be devastated, infectious diseases would increase, and a significant percentage of food and fiber crops would be lost.

But by reducing the amount of pollution in the air and the ground around us, we can help prevent a number of serious illnesses, including:

- **Cardiovascular disease**—The American Heart Association estimates that people living in the most polluted U.S. cities could lose between 1.8 and 3.1 years of life because of exposure to chronic air pollution.
- **Chronic obstructive pulmonary disease (COPD)**—This is a progressive disease characterized by a gradual loss of lung function. The World Health Organization estimates that 42 percent of all cases of COPD worldwide are a result of exposure to workplace dust, fumes, and other forms of indoor and outdoor pollution. And unless cost-effective prevention and management strategies are implemented, the number of cases will continue to increase as the global population ages.
- **Asthma**—Air pollution, usually in combination with indoor environmental conditions and genetic susceptibility, plays a significant role in asthma attacks. Recent studies have shown that the expression of genes associated with asthma is greatly influenced by interaction with the environment. So although asthma is in large part a hereditary immune disorder, your chances of actually having the disease increase greatly with increased exposure to air pollution.
- **Breast cancer**—There have been many studies supporting the association of breast cancer and toxic chemicals, but there are so many variables involved that it has been difficult to prove a direct cause and effect in many cases. Substantial re-

search in the last five years has led scientists to believe that the investigation of environmental pollutants will lead to strategies to reduce breast cancer risk.

SAFEGUARDS AGAINST PESTICIDES

Here are some suggestions on how to keep yourself and your children safer from exposure to pesticides:

- **Minimize personal use and exposure to pesticides in the home and yard.** For instance, I have made it a point not to use pesticides in my own yard and rarely use them in my home. I have had ant problems and have used ant stakes for four to five days to get rid of them. They contain arsenic, but they work and I don't have to keep them around for long periods of time.
- **Use soap to get rid of rodents.** Here in California we have problems with rats and mice getting into car engines and eating through wires and getting into machinery in house basements. If you have the same problem, here's a solution I got from the manager of my car dealership: smear Irish Spring deodorant soap (www.irishspring.com) all around the engine and anywhere else rodents like to go. Apparently they don't like the smell (which is kind of ironic for a deodorant soap . . .). Another way to get rid of rodents is to get a barn owl nest box mounted on top of a stainless steel pole and put it in your yard. It attracts barn owls, which on average eat two thousand rats and mice a year. You can get these boxes at www.owlnestboxes.com or www.hungryowl.org.
- **Use boric acid as an insecticide for control of cockroaches, termites, fire ants, fleas, silverfish, and many other insects.** Boric acid, which can be found in almost any supermarket, hardware store,

or home improvement center, is generally considered to be safe to use in household kitchens to control insects.

- **Make your own pesticides.** Here are a few suggestions:

  - Mix 3 tablespoons of liquid peppermint Castile soap (Dr. Bronner's makes an excellent choice) with 16 ounces of warm water in a spray bottle. Spray directly on insects such as roaches, ants, and spiders.

  - To get rid of cockroaches, get some catnip. In 1999 the American Chemical Association announced that a study had confirmed an old wives' tale— that catnip repels cockroaches. Small sachets of catnip can be left in areas of cockroach activity. Catnip can be also be simmered in a small amount of water to make a "catnip tea." Fill a spray bottle with the "tea," then spray around baseboards and behind counters. Of course, this solution should only be used in homes without cats!

  - Place a few eucalyptus leaves in drawers and closets and around houseplants. Mom always told me insects hate eucalyptus because of its strong odor.

  - Use Amy's Special Mosquito Repellent: My friend Amy places cups of water mixed with distilled vinegar around her plants in her backyard. It attracts the mosquitoes so they don't get you. According to Amy, someone who is usually a mosquito magnet, her Fourth of July celebration in Ohio was at dusk bite free.

For your garden:

- **Bring on the praying mantises, ladybugs, and lacewings** (available at many nurseries); they will get rid of many unwanted pests.
- **Use organic pesticides**, such as Dr. Earth Pro-Active Fruit and Vegetable Insect Spray or Dr. Earth Pro-Active House and Garden Plants Insect

Spray (www.drearth.com); Concern Garden Defense Multi-Purpose Spray (www.arbico-organics .com). Organic pesticides are made from natural substances, are less toxic to humans than commercial brands, and break down quickly into harmless substances.

- **Increase your use of organic fertilizers, mulch, and compost piles**. A few excellent organic fertilizers are Dr. Earth Organic 9 Fruit Tree Fertilizer, Organic 6 Flower Garden Fertilizer and Organic 5 Tomato, Vegetable, and Herb Fertilizer; organic mulch and fertilizer by E.B. Stone (www.ebstone .org), and BioFlora Dry Crumbles (www.bioflora .com). If you feed your plants well (just like Super-Foods for our own bodies), they will thrive and be much less susceptible to pests, fungi, and disease.

Mom Says Love Those Earthworms!

My mother taught me that earthworms are nature's fertilizer factories. They crawl along all day just making fertilizer for your yard. She told me that the more earthworms you have per shovel of earth, the healthier your yard is. When I bought my first home, I was determined to listen to my mother's advice. I talked a patient of mine who owned an earthworm factory into selling me a dump truck-load of dirt teeming with earthworms, which I then spread all around my front and back yards. I have to say, I had the best-looking grass in the neighborhood! And to this day, after every heavy rainstorm when the earthworms are strewn all over the driveway and the walks, I pick them up and throw them back in the grass. They're the cheapest organic fertilizer you can buy!

- **Become a backyard chicken farmer.** You don't have to have a large space to own chickens, and five or six of them will provide fertilizer and pest control for your yard and garden as well as supply you with eggs for the breakfast table. They're also great for getting rid of slugs. Many urban areas are changing zoning laws that once forbade homeowners to have chickens as pets and are allowing up to six chickens per yard. Just make sure there are no roosters in the bunch or you'll have an alarm clock even if you don't want one.

- **Grow your own "be kind to the earth" gardens.** In World Wars I and II, many people here and abroad grew "victory gardens" in their own backyards to reduce the pressure on the public food supply brought on by the war. It's about time we started an updated version, growing as many foods and herbs at home as possible to combat rapidly rising food costs and to help the environment. Food grown in your own garden always tastes better than store bought. It's a great way to spend time with your kids, and it gets you and your children outside getting sunshine (and more vitamin D) and learning to love the environment. It creates a healthy habit and gives you a chance to exercise. Even if you have no yard, you can grow tomatoes (they grow amazingly well indoors). Plant a seed and save the world!

All of us need to remember the saying "Think globally and act locally." We don't really know how the toxins released in our own backyards are affecting the rest of the world. Efforts to investigate the effects of, for instance, organochlorine compounds (hydrocarbon compounds that contain chlorine), including PCBs and pesticides, are difficult because these substances are carried through the air and in the ocean, resulting in substantial exposures even in the Arctic, where these compounds have never even been used! So think of it this way: One person can make a big difference. You may never know exactly how much greening your little part of the world is helping, but I can guarantee it is making the earth healthier for all of us. For the complete Week 2 Daily Planner, see page 292.

◆ MEET TOM ALEXANDER ◆

A Conscientious Man

Ask Tom Alexander what he's changed about his life since he became a follower of SuperHealth, and he'll tell you immediately. "I was always a careful eater," he says, "but now I'm conscientious." What does that mean? "If you're careful," says Alexander, "you might have one piece of cake instead of two or three. If you're conscientious, you say you're not having any cake and you stick to it. It means you do what you say you're going to do almost all the time."

Although he was always a fairly disciplined person, Alexander wasn't always a conscientious eater. Because he grew up on a farm in upstate New York, you might think that he ate well growing up, but the opposite is true.

"The food we ate was a cardiologist's nightmare," he says. "My mom would skim the cream off our fresh milk and pour it into our cereal. The 'jus' from the roast beef we had for dinner would be poured into a glass for us to drink with the meal. If you let that sit out, it would solidify and you could actually see the cholesterol, though we didn't know then that's what it was. Lard was plentiful, and we had butter over everything. Needless to say, by the first time I had my cholesterol checked, it was up around 300."

That's when Alexander became a careful eater. He cut back on fatty foods and stopped eating as many sweets as he had before. He ate salads with iceberg lettuce and a tomato or two. He felt he was making strides toward living a healthier life.

Then he saw Dr. Pratt for a routine checkup and was disturbed to find out he had drusen, tiny yellow or white deposits in the retina of the eye that can indicate the start of macular degeneration, the leading cause of blindness in individuals over age sixty. That's when he became a conscientious eater.

"I follow just what Dr. Pratt told me to do. I eat plenty of leafy green vegetables; in fact, any vegetable with color in it is good for you. I eat broccoli, which is not my favorite. But before, if there was a combination of broccoli, carrots, and cauliflower, I would just ignore the broccoli. Now I look at it and say,

(continued)

'Broccoli, you will be liked!' and I eat it. If there's a choice on a menu between a spinach salad and a Cobb salad, I now order the spinach salad. If you like them both, why not order the one that's better for you? After a while, it becomes a habit."

That's not the only habit Alexander has developed. At seventy-one, he plays tennis once a week, has a treadmill at his home that he's on two or three times a week, and works out with light weights to keep his abs, biceps, and triceps toned. He takes a lutein supplement (for his eyes) and a multivitamin every day. And today his drusen are gone.

"Being conscientious is not all that difficult," he says. "It's about what I choose to eat. It wasn't a question of my eating stuff I didn't like because I thought I'd get better. I just eat more of what I like and a lot less of some of the other stuff that's not so good for you."

5

Step 3: Watch Your Waistline—
Burn Those Calories

*For your basics, see the SuperHealth Food Pyramid,
page 19 (for your bonus see below)*

Week 3 SuperFoods:

Fruit	Tomatoes
Whole grains	Extra virgin olive oil
Yogurt	Honey
Pumpkin	Beans

Why do watching your waistline and burning calories
help promote a longer, healthier life? Because as you
reduce the dangerous fat that settles in your body's
midsection, you decrease your risk of diabetes, high
blood pressure, heart disease, macular degeneration, dementia, Alzheimer's disease, certain kinds of cancer,
and liver dysfunction (it's impossible to be in the Super-
Health zone with an unhealthy liver because your liver
is the main factory for processing the nutrients you consume). You may not be able to change your basic body
type (you can't "will" your fat—no matter how much or
how little—to settle in one part of your body rather
than another, nor can you exercise it all away), but small
changes can make a big difference. The good news in all

of this is that although the propensity toward gaining fat in the "wrong" place may be partially genetic, it's possible to change your shape by losing weight and reducing the size of your waist. In fact, only a 7 to 10 percent reduction in body weight and/or a two-inch reduction in waist size (which are realistic and attainable goals) helps reduce your risk for many chronic diseases such as diabetes, macular degeneration, high blood pressure, and cancer.

REDUCE YOUR TOXIC WAIST

In the 1980s health professionals began using a formula called the Body Mass Index (BMI) to calculate obesity. Dividing a person's weight by the square of his or her height became the international standard for obesity measurement (to find your BMI, see page 340). A normal BMI is between 19 and 24.9; people with a BMI of below 19 are judged to be underweight; those with a BMI of 25 to 29.9 are overweight; and those with a BMI of 30 or more are considered to be obese.

BMI does not directly measure percentage of body fat, but it provides a more accurate measure of overweight and obesity than relying on weight alone. The problem with BMI is that it can lead to the misclassification of some people; for instance, an athlete with a high amount of muscle mass might have a BMI greater than 25, but that doesn't necessarily mean he or she is overweight. A thin person may believe that all is well because of his or her BMI of 21; however, that reading doesn't take body shape into account. And it turns out that body shape is very important.

That's why the Japanese are so concerned about the size of their waistlines, and why we should be, too. In early 2008 the country of Japan began a campaign to get its citizenry to lose weight. As part of that effort, companies and local government were required to measure the waistlines of Japanese people between the ages of forty and seventy-four as part of their annual checkups.

Those who exceed government standards (33.5 inches for men and 35.4 inches for women—remember that most Japanese are smaller than most Americans; standards are different around the world) and don't lose weight within three months are given dieting guidance and are to receive reeducation if they don't lose enough weight after six months.

While this kind of government intervention may seem foreign to Westerners, it does underscore what health professionals worldwide are seeing as one of the most significant guidelines to your ongoing health, vitality, and longevity: the circumference of your waist. In other words, if you can whittle down your waistline (in the United States the suggested standards are thirty-five inches for women and forty inches for men), you'll be making major strides toward living in the Super-Health zone, decreasing your risk for diabetes, macular degeneration, metabolic syndrome, high blood pressure, and atherosclerosis (which leads to increased risk for coronary heart disease and stroke).

If you are a woman and your waist circumference is more than thirty-five inches, and/or your waist-to-hip ratio (WHR)—waist circumference divided by hip circumference (turn to page 342 for the full formula)—is greater than 0.8, or if you're a man with a waist circumference of more than forty inches and/or a WHR of more than 0.9, you have an increased risk for the development of obesity-related factors including impaired glucose tolerance, insulin resistance, type 2 diabetes, high blood pressure, cataracts, macular degeneration (causing loss of functional vision), high triglycerides, low HDL, and high total cholesterol (all risk factors for cardiovascular disease), some types of cancer, and elevated inflammatory markers such as C-reactive protein (meaning you have too much inflammation in your body, which can lead to most, if not all, of the diseases of modern man).

Although waist circumference and WHR are not perfect screening modalities for every body type (the same standards apply whether you are five feet three or six feet tall), in general they do a good job of relating our body measurements to risk for disease.

In reality, you don't need a tape measure or even a scale to tell if your WHR (known in some irreverent circles as the butt-to-belly ratio) is where it should be. Stand up straight, feet together, and put your chin to your chest; if you can't see your feet, it might be time to add some SuperFoods into your diet, start exercising ten to fifteen minutes a day, and make some positive changes in your life. If you do want to keep track, make it fun. Remember how as a kid you used to anxiously await your newest height measurement on the garage wall? You were thrilled with yourself for reaching a new goal. Give yourself the same pat on the back for every pound and every inch you lose.

ARE YOU AN APPLE OR A PEAR?

If your hips are wider than your shoulders and your WHR is below 0.8, you are a "pear" and you store most of your weight in your hips and thighs. If you're pear shaped, you're more prone to problems like varicose veins and cellulite. Pear-shaped women have fewer androgens in their bodies (male hormones that, among other things, increase bone mass), and weaker estrogen at menopause, which makes them more susceptible to osteoporosis.

If your WHR is above 0.8, you're most likely an "apple" and your weight distribution is centered at your middle. Many men are apples—think beer bellies (remember, there's no such thing as a salad belly). Women are more prone to develop the apple shape after menopause, which may be because that's when women produce fewer female hormones, such as estrogen, so their shape tends to become more "male."

The truth is you don't want to be an apple or a pear. You want to be strong and lean, and not bulging out in front, in back, or side to side.

What you want to reduce is what is called visceral fat,

the kind of fat that develops around your middle (commonly called belly fat). You might not realize it, but there are two types of fat in your body. The fat that is located just under the skin is called subcutaneous fat. Fat that is found in the abdomen and surrounding vital organs is called visceral fat; it is this type of fat that causes the most health concerns—and here are a few reasons why:

- Visceral fat does more than just take up space. Scientists now believe that fat cells secrete hormones and other substances. In fact, some scientists now call fat an "endocrine organ," comparing it to glands such as the thyroid and the pituitary that also release hormones straight into the bloodstream.
- Visceral fat can be metabolized by the liver, which turns it into cholesterol that circulates in the blood, collects in the arteries, and forms artery-clogging plaque. Visceral fat also releases leptin, a hormone that communicates the degree of hunger to the brain in order to help control appetite (and secondarily body fat). Scientists had hoped that leptin might help solve the obesity problem, but it turns out that most obese people are resistant to its effects.
- Visceral fat cells produce a hormone called adiponectin, which makes the body more sensitive to insulin. Logically it would seem that the fatter you were, the more adiponectin you would produce, which would help utilize insulin. Unfortunately, although no one knows why, the opposite is true. The heavier you are, the less adiponectin you produce and the less sensitive to insulin you become, and the more insulin you require. Remember, a SuperHealth goal is to decrease your body's insulin requirements.
- Visceral fat secretes pro-inflammatory chemicals such as TNFα (tumor necrosis factor), which (among other things) decreases our muscles' ability to regulate blood sugar levels.

In an average person about 10 percent of body fat is visceral, while 90 percent is subcutaneous. In a very obese person that ratio changes to about 25:75. Therefore, it stands to reason that shrinking as much visceral fat as possible is one of the best ways to ensure a longer, healthier life, and following the SuperHealth plan is one of the best ways to reduce both the visceral and subcutaneous fat that make up abdominal girth.

In this chapter we'll be focusing on nutrient-dense foods that can help you lose that "belly fat" and on beginning to add physical activity into your daily routine, both of which will help you to:

- Prevent cardiovascular disease
- Prevent metabolic syndrome: a cluster of metabolic risk factors including insulin resistance (more and more insulin required to force blood sugar into our cells), hypertension (high blood pressure), elevated cholesterol/triglycerides (fats that increase our risk for cardiovascular disease), high blood sugar levels, and high levels of inflammation, all leading to increased risk for diabetes, heart attacks, stroke, dementia, cancer, and premature death.
- Reduce coronary calcium: Belly fat is not only a risk factor for coronary heart disease incidents and mortality, but it is also a marker for early subclinical atherosclerosis (hardening of the arteries) in people of all ages. The bigger the waist, the more coronary calcium (plaque) you're likely to have, and the bigger the risk for future cardiac events.

SUPERHEALTH WAIST WATCHER PLAN

In addition to the foods introduced in the SuperHealth Plans for Weeks 1 and 2 (especially berries and green leafy vegetables), this week focuses on eight specifically waist-friendly foods that help reduce your belly fat and control your blood sugar, which affects insulin production and therefore reduces your probability of developing diabetes. These are fruit, whole grains, yogurt, pumpkin, tomatoes, extra virgin olive oil, honey, and beans.

We start off with fruit and whole grains because of their dietary fiber content. Increasing the amount of fiber in your diet is one of the best methods of reducing your waist. Fiber is great at regulating blood sugar, because fiber (in addition to aiding in the digestion of food and the elimination of waste) helps to slow down the rate at which you absorb the carbohydrates you eat. If you're not absorbing the carbohydrates so quickly, you'll end up losing inches.

I recommend the following fiber goals:

- 45 grams of fiber a day for men
- 32 grams of fiber a day for women

This may be more fiber than you're used to eating, and it will seem daunting at first—a serving of a high-fiber food such as flaxseed has only 4 grams of fiber. But I'll give you a plan for adding more fiber to this week. You can achieve your goal by eating whole fruits instead of drinking fruit juices; choosing whole grain cereals with at least 3 grams of fiber per serving; boosting the fiber content of any cereal by adding oat bran, wheat germ or wheat bran, or flaxseed meal; eating brown rice and whole grain bread (with at least 3 grams of fiber per slice) instead of white rice and white bread; snacking on raw vegetables (e.g., broccoli and asparagus); consuming green leafy vegetables like spinach, Swiss chard, and collard greens; adding legumes to your diet; and including a number of meals each week that are made with beans instead of meat. (Turn to page 264 for a list of the best choices of high-fiber foods.)

Many studies have shown that a high-fiber diet is an important part of reaching and maintaining optimum weight goals. Not only does it help reduce blood sugar levels; it also decreases calorie intake and promotes weight loss because it makes you feel full, and that stops you from eating too much.

> ### Feeling Full? Give It a Minute (or Twenty)
>
> Fiber is great for helping you feel full—but don't depend solely on your whole grain to tell you when to stop eating. It takes about twenty minutes for your stomach to send the message to your brain: "I'm full. Stop eating." So eat slowly, and after you finish your first servings, wait for a few minutes to see if you're really still hungry.

Fruit

Recommended amount: minimum of 3 to 5 servings a day, including berries most days. Servings equal:

- ½ cup chopped fruit (½ baseball)
- ½ cup 100% fruit juice (whole fruit is best, but for the sake of convenience, juice is acceptable); my favorites are orange juice with pulp, pomegranate juice, Concord grape juice, and blueberry juice.
- 1 medium piece of fruit (1 baseball)
- 2 tablespoons (1 shot glass) raisins or 3 to 7 prunes

Along with the many vitamins and polyphenols that fruits provide, they are also an excellent source of dietary fiber, which is the reason they (along with whole grains) are included in this particular step.

Apples (and their sidekick, pears) are a particularly good source of fiber. I eat at least one apple every day. But apples and pears aren't the only fruits that are good sources of fiber. Here are some other suggestions:

Fruit	Servings	Grams of Fiber
Raspberries	1 cup (1 baseball)	8.4 grams
Blackberries	1 cup (1 baseball)	7.6 grams
Persimmons	1 large (1 baseball)	6.1 grams
Apple	1 medium (1 baseball)	5.7 grams
Kiwi	2 medium	5 grams
Avocado	½ cup (½ baseball)	4.2 grams
Pear	1 medium (1 baseball)	4 grams
Blueberries	1 cup (1 baseball)	3.9 grams
Strawberries	1 cup (1 baseball)	3.5 grams
Orange	1 medium (1 baseball)	3.4 grams
Figs	2 medium	3.3 grams
Dates	5–6 pitted	3 grams
Papaya	1 cup cubes (1 baseball)	2.5 grams
Nectarine	1 medium (1 baseball)	2.3 grams
Peach	1 medium (1 baseball)	2.3 grams
Applesauce—Tree Top	½ cup (½ baseball)	2 grams
Applesauce—Mott's Organic Unsweetened	½ cup (½ baseball)	1 gram

And if you're looking for fiber sources from veggies, here are my top recommendations:

Vegetable	Servings	Grams of Fiber
Peas (dried)	½ cup (½ baseball)	8 grams
Peas (cooked)	½ cup (½ baseball)	5 grams
Winter squash (cooked)	½ cup (½ baseball)	3 grams
Bell pepper	1 medium	3 grams
Broccoli (cooked)	½ cup (½ baseball)	2.4 grams
Green beans (cooked)	½ cup (½ baseball)	2 grams
Brussels sprouts (cooked)	½ cup (½ baseball)	2 grams
Carrots (cooked)	½ cup (½ baseball)	1.8 grams
Kale (cooked)	½ cup (½ baseball)	1.8 grams
Cauliflower (cooked)	½ cup (½ baseball)	1.7 grams
Asparagus (cooked)	½ cup (½ baseball)	1.5 grams

Don't Skip the Skin

Much of the fiber in fruit is in the skin, especially when it comes to apples, pears, peaches, and nectarines. So wash the fruit well, then eat the whole fruit with the skin, and get the full benefit of the fiber.

Absolute musts: If there's only one fruit you add for the week, or if you're traveling and can't control your diet, my recommendation is at least one apple or pear a day and one serving of berries.

Whole Grains

Recommended amount: 10 grams of whole grain fiber a day (which means that 10 of your 32 or 45 dietary fiber grams a day should come from whole grains). For instance, 1¼ cups of Post Shredded Wheat 'N Bran gives you 8 grams fiber. Add 2 tablespoons of ground flaxseed to this at breakfast (4 grams of fiber) and you've met your quota. You'll find a more complete list of high-fiber foods and their gram counts on page 264. There's a bakery here in California that makes a delicious whole grain bread that has 12 grams of fiber per slice (www.julianbakery.com). Make a sandwich of that bread, and you're more than set for the day at a whopping 24 grams.

When grains are processed or refined—to make white bread or white rice, for instance—the bran (outer layer) and the germ (inner layer) are stripped away, along with their many natural nutrients, antioxidants, and phytochemicals. To be certain that the foods you're buying actually contain whole grains, make sure the list of ingredients on the label says "whole," and not just "hearty" or "multi" grain. Choose breads and cereals with a fiber content of at least 3 grams per serving.

Here are some suggested SuperHealth high-fiber whole grains:

Grain	Amount	Grams of Fiber
Pearled barley	¼ cup uncooked	8 grams
Arrowhead Mills Organic Stone Ground Buckwheat Flour	¼ cup	6 grams
Quaker Oat Bran Hot Cereal	½ cup	6 grams
Orville Redenbacher's Gourmet Popping Corn	3 tablespoons	6 grams
Bob's Red Mill Rolled Oats Whole Grain Hot Cereal	½ cup	5 grams
Bob's Red Mill 100% Whole Grain Cornmeal	¼ cup	5 grams
365 Organic Whole Wheat Shells www.wholefoodsmarket.com	¾ cup	5 grams
Trader Joe's Organic Whole Wheat Spaghetti	2 ounces	5 grams
Bob's Red Mill Rolled Triticale (a hybrid of rye and wheat) www.bobsredmill.com	¼ cup	4 grams
Bob's Red Mill Whole Ground Flaxseed Meal	2 tablespoons	4 grams
Arrowhead Mills Organic Stone Ground Whole Wheat Flour www.arrowheadmills.com	½ cup	4 grams
Arrowhead Mills Organic Stone Ground Rye Flour	¼ cup	4 grams
Arrowhead Mills Organic Stone Ground Spelt Flour (a type of wheat but with a nuttier flavor)	¼ cup	4 grams
Arrowhead Mills Organic Stone Ground Kamut Flour (a high-protein wheat variety)	¼ cup	4 grams
Bob's Red Mill Rice Bran	2 tablespoons	3 grams

(continued)

Grain	Amount	Grams of Fiber
Bob's Red Mill 100% Stone Ground Amaranth Flour	¼ cup	3 grams
Arrowhead Mills Organic Stone Ground Millet Flour	¼ cup	3 grams
Arrowhead Mills Organic Stone Ground Yellow Corn Meal	¼ cup	3 grams
Lundberg Eco-Farmed Long-Grain Brown Rice (www.lundberg.com)	¼ cup	3 grams
Quinoa	¼ cup uncooked	2.5 grams
Kretschmer Toasted Wheat Germ	2 tablespoons	2 grams
365 Organic Long-Grain Brown Rice	¼ cup	2 grams

Absolute musts: If there's only one whole grain you add for the week, or if you're traveling and can't control your diet, my recommendation is 2 tablespoons of ground flaxseed, wheat bran, oat bran, or corn bran, which you can sprinkle on oatmeal, cereal, or yogurt, or use in smoothies, pancakes, muffins, and quickbreads. I put some in a plastic container and stick it in my suitcase when I'm traveling. As an added benefit, 4 grams of whole grain bran a day is all you need to statistically decrease your risk of atherosclerosis (hardening of the arteries), which we now know is related to having a big belly.

Yogurt (Nonfat)

Recommended amount: 1 to 2 cups (1 to 2 baseballs) most days

Sidekicks: kefir (a creamy drink made from fermented cow's milk), soy yogurt

Many of the health benefits of yogurt are due to the

power of probiotics. Probiotics are live organisms, healthful bacteria that are often added to yogurt. These bacteria perform biological functions that are important to our survival. Probiotic means "for life," as opposed to antibiotic, which is "against life" (antibiotics kill bacteria). Look for nonfat yogurt (organic when possible) that contains the National Yogurt Association "live active cultures" seal on the container. Some of my favorites are Cascade Fresh Fat Free Yogurt, Whole Foods 365 Organic Nonfat Yogurt, Wallaby Organic Nonfat Yogurt, Alta Dena Nonfat Yogurt, Brown Cow All Natural Nonfat Yogurt, Horizon Organic Fat Free Yogurt, and Stonyfield Farm Organic Nonfat Yogurt.

It turns out that the probiotics found in yogurt are good for your gastrointestinal health and for weight loss as well. Think of probiotics as your own internal weight-loss factory. A healthy GI system metabolizes calories more efficiently than one that is not so healthy. Studies have shown that healthy bacteria aid weight loss; for instance, in a 2008 study conducted at Stanford University, obese patients who took probiotics after undergoing gastric bypass surgery lost more weight than patients who had the surgery but did not take the supplements. Scientists have also learned that healthy lean individuals have totally different bacterial flora in their GI tract than folks who are overweight and eat a lot of white starch and fat. When the GI tracts of thin mice were sterilized and the bacteria from fat mice were transplanted into their systems, the thin mice got fat without consuming any more calories than they usually did. What that means to you is that if you "transplant" good flora into your own GI tract by consuming yogurt daily, your gut will react like that of a healthy-weight individual and begin to help you lose weight. It's an easy step to take to get you on your way to SuperHealth.

In addition to probiotics, some of the benefits of yogurt are enhanced by prebiotics, which essentially are food for probiotics. Prebiotics are not digestible, but they selectively interact with our intestinal microbiota. Stonyfield Farm yogurts contain inulin (a prebiotic fiber). Four SuperFoods you can add to your diet to provide nourishment for probiotics are honey, blueberries, raisins, and tea (honey's unique carbohydrate composition primarily includes the monosaccharides glucose and fructose, but also about 5 percent oligosaccharides, which are known to support the growth of probiotics). So go to town with a snack-time treat of raisins, or nonfat organic yogurt mixed with fresh blueberries, served with a refreshing cup of green tea sweetened with honey (less than a teaspoon).

Try My Special Green Tea Drink

Steep two green tea bags in 4 ounces of hot water for about 3 minutes. If you squeeze the tea bags dry you get twice the polyphenol content out of it (so you now have the polypherol content of about four cups of green tea in the 4 ounces of water). Add 4 to 8 ounces of organic soymilk (for example, Silk or Kirkland [Costco]) and 1 teaspoon of dark (preferably buckwheat) honey. Now we're talking SuperHealth!

Absolute musts: If there's only one yogurt dish you add for the week for watching your waistline, or if you're traveling and can't control your diet, my recommendation is to make this quick, healthy breakfast: Mix 1 cup of nonfat yogurt with fresh fruit—berries, sliced oranges, or whatever is in season—and sprinkle with some wheat germ, crushed nuts, and a drizzle of honey. If you can't get your yogurt serving in, get DanActive Immunity, a probiotic dairy drink by Dannon (90 calories—three sips and you're done), or you can use Sustenex, a probiotic capsule with bacteria that survive and thrive in your digestive tract (available at most drugstores and health food stores or at www.sustenex.com).

Pumpkin

Recommended amount: ½ cup (½ baseball), five to seven days a week

Sidekicks: carrots, butternut squash, sweet potatoes, orange bell peppers

Not only is this group of foods noted for its fiber content and bountiful supply of vitamins and minerals; it is also loaded with carotenoids. Carotenoids are a group of six hundred to seven hundred compounds; the better-known ones are alpha-carotene and beta-carotene, beta-cryptoxanthin, lycopene, lutein, and zeaxanthin, which produce the red, yellow, and orange colors found in many fruits and vegetables. Carotenoids help to preserve muscle mass, and if you're losing weight, you don't want to lose muscle; you just want to lose fat. So independent of whether you work out or not, there is a positive relationship between carotenoid intake and muscle mass and muscle strength.

Recent studies have also shown that serum carotenoids are inversely associated with type 2 diabetes and impaired glucose metabolism—meaning that the more carotenoids you eat, the better your blood sugar is regulated and the lower your risk of developing diabetes. They are also potent antioxidants and may play a protective role against the development of chronic diseases including cancers, cardiovascular disease, and inflammatory diseases.

Sweet potatoes are good simply steamed and served with a drizzle of melted Smart Balance or other buttery spread and a sprinkle of cinnamon or nutmeg; winter squash (such as butternut, buttercup, and Hubbard) can be prepared by cutting them in half, drizzling on a bit of honey and a sprinkle of black pepper, and baking at 350° F until the flesh is soft. Pumpkin smoothies are delicious—you can find a recipe on page 286.

Absolute musts: If there's only one pumpkin item you add for the week, or if you're traveling and can't control your diet, my recommendation is one 8-ounce glass of carrot juice most days.

Tomatoes

Recommended amount: 1 serving of cooked or processed tomatoes, such as 1 to 2 tablespoons of tomato paste (see page 271 for more suggestions) or sidekicks listed below, a day, and multiple servings a week of fresh tomatoes

Sidekicks: watermelon, pink grapefruit, red-fleshed papayas, Japanese persimmons, strawberry guavas

Tomatoes (and sidekicks) are another great source of carotenoids, one of which is the powerful antioxidant lycopene. Like pumpkin, tomatoes help control blood sugar and help preserve muscle mass. Besides being a staple in every weight-loss program, tomatoes have been found to help prevent prostate and pancreatic cancer and cardiovascular disease. They also have been shown to be an effective blood thinner, good for anyone who is susceptible to blood clot formation. Look for low-sodium tomato juice (and if that's too bland for you, add a dash of hot sauce, a squeeze of lemon, or a touch of Mrs. Dash or Kirkland No-Salt Seasoning). Lycopene actually is more available after cooking or processing, so don't forget to use canned tomato paste in sauces, soups, and stews.

Absolute musts: If there's only one tomato serving you add for the week, or if you're traveling and can't control your diet, my recommendation is one 8-ounce glass of low-sodium tomato juice or R.W. Knudsen Very Veggie Low Sodium Vegetable Cocktail a day.

Extra Virgin Olive Oil (EVOO)

Recommended amount: 1 to 2 tablespoons most days
Sidekick: canola oil

If you want to help insulin do its job (and you do), reduce your intake of saturated animal fats and trans fats, which are found in many processed foods. But don't cut out fats altogether—instead go for polyunsaturated and monounsaturated fats found in nuts and seeds, wild salmon, and first-cold-pressed extra virgin olive oil

(EVOO). Cold-pressing is a chemical-free process using only pressure, which produces a higher quality of olive oil that is naturally lower in acidity. It also maximizes the phytonutrient content of the oil.

Remember, however, that olive oil is a fat. It has 120 calories per tablespoon. If you eat too much of it, you will gain weight. For most people it's best used as a substitute for other less healthy fats, such as butter.

Honey

Recommended amount: 1 to 2 teaspoons, multiple times a week (buckwheat honey, if possible—the darker the honey, the more polyphenols it contains)

Honey helps to maintain optimal blood sugar levels (the flavonoids in the honey help our body regulate blood sugar—the darker the honey, the more flavonoids it contains). Honey is also helpful for maintaining energy levels and restoring muscle recovery after exercise. It also helps reduce oxidative stress—as the waist gets bigger, the number of pro-inflammatory chemicals goes up, the number of free radicals goes up, and you're now in a state of oxidative stress. All the diseases related to a big waist are tied into the imbalance of too many free radicals and not enough antioxidants; therefore, you want your diet to include foods that reduce oxidative stress.

When I was growing up we never had table sugar in the house. We used honey in and on everything. In fact, my mom would give us honeycombs and we would chew on the wax. Honey is more than just a sweetener for your tea. It is one of the oldest medicines known to man, and it contains at least 181 different substances that have made it useful in the treatment of ailments from respiratory disease, skin ulcers, wounds, and gastrointestinal diseases to eczema, psoriasis, and dandruff. It has a high level of oligosaccharides (food for health-promoting probiotic bacteria), which increase the number of "good" bacteria in the colon. To get more honey in your diet, use it for more than just a beverage sweetener (honey also boosts the antioxidant capacity of your blood, just like blueberries). Drizzle a teaspoon into plain yogurt to sweeten. Or you can make a delicious honey-mustard salad dressing by mixing two tablespoons each of honey and Dijon mustard, a drizzle of lemon juice, and ¼ cup extra virgin olive oil. Serve on peppery greens such as arugula.

Beans

Recommended amount: at least four ½ cup (½ baseball) servings a week

Sidekicks: All legumes are included in this SuperFood category; some of the most popular and readily available varieties are pinto beans, kidney beans, navy beans, great Northern beans, lima beans, garbanzo beans (chickpeas), lentils, string beans (or green beans), sugar snap peas, and green peas

The abundant soluble fiber in beans works hard to stabilize blood sugar levels. Beans provide the steady, slow-burning energy that keeps glucose levels well regulated. A stable blood sugar is helpful not only for controlling diabetes but also for weight management. Beans provide bulk with minimal calories. They fill you up, minimizing hunger and maintaining high energy levels throughout the day. Here are some examples of the fiber content of beans:

SuperFood	Serving Size	Grams of Fiber
Black beans	1 cup cooked	15 grams
Lentils	1 cup cooked	15 grams
Pinto beans	1 cup cooked	14 grams
Green peas	1 cup cooked	9 grams

Beans also offer a healthy source of protein. Just 1 cup of lentils provides 17 grams of protein with only .75 grams of fat. Two ounces of extra-lean trimmed sirloin steak has the same amount of protein but six times the fat. Lentils are quick to cook—they don't require presoaking like many other beans—and are very versatile. Add a bit of curry powder to give them an Indian flavor or some chopped garlic, celery, and olive oil for a more traditional take. If you're buying canned beans, look for low-sodium or no-salt-added beans, or rinse the beans in cold water, which will remove much of the salt.

Week 3: Watch Your Waistline Daily Food Planner

The chart below is an example of how you can add waist-watching foods to your SuperHealth program. It shows you how to get more waist-watching friendly foods into your diet—but it doesn't mean these are the only foods you should eat for the week. They are just suggestions; feel free to mix and match foods and days to your heart's content.

	Food Suggestion	Daily Servings
Day 1	Unsweetened applesauce	½ cup (½ baseball)
	Ground flaxseed	2 tablespoons (1 shot glass)
	Yogurt	1 cup (1 baseball)
	Carrots	½ cup (½ baseball)
	Tomato	1 medium (1 baseball)
	Lentils (cooked)	½ cup (½ baseball)
	Buckwheat honey	1 to 2 tablespoons (1 to 2 shot glasses)
	EVOO	2 tablespoons (1 shot glass)
Day 2	Avocado	½ cup (½ baseball)
	Wheat bran	2 tablespoons (1 shot glass)
	Yogurt (soy)	1 cup (1 baseball)
	Pumpkin	½ cup (½ baseball)
	Tomato paste	2 tablespoons (1 shot glass)
	Chickpeas	½ cup (½ baseball)
	Buckwheat honey	1 to 2 tablespoons (1 to 2 shot glasses)
	EVOO	2 tablespoons (1 shot glass)
Day 3	Blueberries	1 cup (1 baseball)
	Whole grain bread	2 slices

(continued)

	Food Suggestion	Daily Servings
Day 3 *(cont.)*	Yogurt	1 cup (1 baseball)
	Sweet potato	½ cup (½ baseball)
	Pink grapefruit	½ grapefruit
	String beans	1 cup (1 baseball)
	Buckwheat honey	1 to 2 tablespoons (1 to 2 shot glasses)
	EVOO	2 tablespoons (1 shot glass)
Day 4	Orange	1 medium (1 baseball)
	Bran cereal	1 cup (1 baseball)
	Carrots	½ cup (½ baseball)
	Tomato	1 medium (1 baseball)
	EVOO	2 tablespoons (1 shot glass)
Day 5	Pear	1 medium (1 baseball)
	Quinoa (cooked)	½ cup (½ baseball)
	Yogurt (soy)	1 cup (1 baseball)
	Butternut squash	½ cup (½ baseball)
	Tomato	1 medium (1 baseball)
	Kidney beans (cooked)	½ cup (½ baseball)
	Buckwheat honey	1 to 2 tablespoons (1 to 2 shot glasses)
	EVOO	2 tablespoons (1 shot glass)
Day 6	Strawberries	1 cup (1 baseball)
	Brown rice (cooked)	½ cup (½ baseball)
	Yogurt	1 cup (1 baseball)
	Orange bell pepper	½ cup (½ baseball)
	Watermelon	1 cup cubed (1 baseball)
	Buckwheat honey	1 to 2 tablespoons (1 to 2 shot glasses)
	EVOO	2 tablespoons (1 shot glass)
Day 7	Nectarine	1 medium (1 baseball)
	Ground flaxseed	2 tablespoons (1 shot glass)
	Pumpkin	½ cup (½ baseball)
	Tomato	1 medium (1 baseball)
	Green peas	½ cup (½ baseball)
	Buckwheat honey	1 to 2 tablespoons (1 to 2 shot glasses)
	EVOO	2 tablespoons (1 shot glass)

BURN THOSE CALORIES

I know what the ultimate American fantasy is. It's not Prince or Princess Charming riding up on a white horse. It's not a tropical vacation with perfect weather, bikini-clad women, and naturally tanned cabana boys. It's not even winning the lottery. Here's the top fantasy of all time: exercise in a bottle. Drink a six-pack of exercise, get a six-pack of abs. All you ever have to do is walk to the fridge and back and you'll be fit, attractive, and healthy for life.

Sorry, folks. Exercise is not something that comes in a bottle, a pill, or a syringe. It comes from your mind, your muscles, and your metabolism, and you've got to get all three working if you want to attain SuperHealth (or any kind of health at all).

There are dozens of reasons exercise is good for you, but here are my top six:

- Exercise helps you lose and maintain ideal weight, which extends your life span and decreases your risk for chronic disease; almost all modern diseases are related in one way or another to being over-weight or obese. The best diet in the world is not going to do it on its own. You cannot get into the SuperHealth zone without burning calories.
- Exercise helps control your blood sugar, which in turn gives you the best chance of avoiding most of the chronic diseases associated with aging.
- Exercise helps prevent cardiovascular disease and cancer (the major causes of death in the United States).
- Exercise helps preserve the senses, especially eyesight and cognitive abilities (brain health).
- Exercise helps maintain healthy bones and muscles so as to prevent falls, fractures, and poor posture.
- Exercise helps you look and feel your best. Physical activity produces endorphins (feel-good hormones) in your brain, which improve your mood,

decrease your risk of depression, and actually pump up your motivation to do more physical activity.

Our ancient ancestors did not have to worry about exercise—there was no such thing as "exercise" as we think of it today; there was simply survival. They needed to be able to hunt game and carry it back to the rest of the tribe. They needed to be able to walk long distances in the face of climate change and to withstand drought or famine. They were forced to be fit. Our ancestors were tough and strong—but they also had a much shorter life span. We're trying to get our bodies to last one hundred years (if not more), and that's a lot of potential wear and tear. But we're not built like fragile china, meant to sit on a shelf lest we be broken into pieces. We're machines, meant to be well maintained and used every day to keep us in the best working order. In the twenty-first-century Western world, we have to put conscious effort into getting enough movement into our daily lives to keep us strong and healthy, both mentally and physically.

But that is not as difficult as you think. The Super-Health Exercise Plan shows you ways to exercise without having to be a fanatic about it, in small chunks that blow away the persistent "I don't have enough time to exercise" excuse. For instance, when I was growing up, my parents installed a pull-up bar in one of our hallways. Every time I walked by that bar, I'd stop and do a few pull-ups and eventually I set the high school record for being able to perform the most number of pull-ups. I didn't have to go to the gym to accomplish this feat, and it cost my parents next to nothing to install the bar.

Many people think they don't like to exercise—until they start doing it. For some reason many of my patients have a mental block about how much of a chore it will be to exercise, or how intimidating (with visions of perfectly toned twenty-year-olds on the next treadmill) or time-consuming it will be. Before you can adjust your fitness aptitude, you have to adjust your fitness attitude. You can be fit and healthy even if you never step on a treadmill in a gym in your life. One young woman I know started out by walking for fifteen or twenty minutes a day. During her walk she would run for thirty seconds (she timed herself with a stopwatch). Every few days she added another thirty-second running interval. Eventually she was running for the whole twenty minutes. So you see, it takes only thirty seconds to get started!

So, to begin . . .

If you are not used to exercising, here are few ways to get you started:

- **Walk the walk:** This is the most basic, the easiest, and probably the most important step you can take (pun intended) toward getting into the Super-Health Fitness zone. Walking is the most common form of physical activity, it costs nothing, it can be done anywhere, and it reconnects us with the environment (which is where our genes would love us to be), with the sounds and smells of nature. We walk every day as part of everything we do. Get a pedometer (at most sporting goods stores or by checking out various brands at http://walking.about.com) and aim for 10,000 steps a day (which is about five miles). You may find out you're already doing quite a bit of walking, and if you're active, you'll be up to about 10,000 steps a day anyway. If the pedometer says that you're getting under 5,000 steps a day, then you're living a sedentary lifestyle. If the pedometer says that you're getting from 7,500 to 10,000 steps, then you're somewhat active. If it tells you that you're getting 10,000 to 12,500 steps, then you're leading an active lifestyle. And if you're getting 12,500 or more, that's even better—you're very active.

  But what if you aren't getting 10,000 steps into your day? A reasonable goal for most people is to increase average daily steps each week by 500 per day until you can easily average 10,000 per day. For example: If you currently average 3,000 steps each day, your goal for Week 1 is 3,500 steps each day. Your Week 2 goal is 4,000 steps each day. Continue to increase each week and you should be averaging 10,000 steps by the end of fourteen weeks.

Where do you find those extra steps without taking enormous amounts of extra time? Easy. Begin with 15 minutes of walking four to five days during the first week. Walk the kids, walk the grandkids, walk your parents, walk your dog. Stop taking technology shortcuts. Instead of sending an e-mail or picking up the phone, walk to chat with your office colleagues. Instead of using the remote, get up and change the channel. Park your car a little farther away from the store or the building and walk a little longer. And don't remove your pedometer when you do SuperHealth's exercise program—the movements you're making when you exercise count too, and they may even count for more than the pedometer registers if you're working up a sweat. If you do all of these things, 10,000 steps a day won't be unrealistic at all. In terms of speed, the ultimate goal is to walk 100 steps per minute for at least 30 minutes five to seven times a week (you can break the 30 minutes down into 10 minutes at a time).

- **Dr. Steve's Power Stairs Workout:** It's easy—all you need is a stairway somewhere in your home or office that you can freely walk up and down. Start with a 1- to 2-minute climb, and build up to 10 to 15 minutes. When you can walk up and down easily for 15 minutes, walk up and down faster and faster (hold on to the rail to avoid a fall—even I usually do this). This exercise gives you maximum bang for the buck, as in a small space of time you are getting strength, power, and aerobics training. Do this two to four times a week. It builds cardiorespiratory health quickly and helps to add quad strength (those big muscles in the front of the thighs). Step up the stairs on your toes if possible (it builds calf strength and will be easier on those aching old knees). When I am stressed out in my office, I go "run the stairs" for 5 minutes. It does wonders for my fight-or-flight response—there are no cave bears in my office, just too many patients for the time allowed, too many phone calls, and too much paperwork.

- **Heel to Fanny:** Stand on stairs or an elevated area (this can be done on a flat surface as well), and hold on to the railing or the wall keeping your knees together. The left leg remains straight. With your right leg beginning in a straight position, bring your right heel to your fanny. You may not be able to touch your fanny, but take it as far as you can and hold it there for 2 seconds, then let it down slowly. Do 3 sets of 10 with each leg, three to four days a week. This builds strength in the hamstrings, those big muscles in the backs of the thighs.

- **Sit-up/Crunch:** Lie on your back with your knees bent and your feet flat on the floor in front of you. Lie on an exercise mat or carpet rather than a hard floor to prevent back strain. Your feet should be as wide apart as your hips. Place your arms crossed on your chest and keep your chin pointing upward. Curl up and forward so that your head, neck, and shoulder blades lift off the floor. Pause for a count of one, then slowly lower your shoulder blades, neck, and head to the starting position. Start off by doing 3 sets of 10, three days a week.

The combination of exercises above will increase your cardiovascular fitness (heart and lungs) and also begin to strengthen your abs and those all-important leg muscles, which you will be depending on to help achieve SuperHealth. Strong leg muscles will help you prevent falls, frailty, and disability and maintain independence as you age.

In the car or at your desk at work:

- **Isometric Curl:** Hold on to the back of the steering wheel (while at a stop sign or signal) at the five o'clock and seven o'clock positions with your palms facing toward you and your arms bent. This can also be done by grabbing the edge of a desk or table, palms facing up, elbows at your sides, shoulders down. The idea is to attempt to bring your hands up toward your shoulders (you won't actually be able to do it—the point is to get the resistance). Hold the position for ten to twenty seconds and repeat 10 times using both arms. This helps to tone the biceps and the front part of the shoulder muscles. For maximum benefit, vary the amount of arm bend slightly for each rep, as this strengthens the muscle at varying degrees of use. Make sure to keep your shoulders down and back. Do this two to three times a week.

- **Isometric Extension:** Again, this is a nonmovement form of strengthening. This time you're pushing against the steering wheel, desk, or any other immobile surface, with the heel of your hand and your fingers pointing down. Try to extend or straighten your arms, using your body weight to resist. Hold the position for 10 to 20 seconds and repeat 10 times using both arms. This helps to tone the triceps (backs of the arms). Do this two to four times a week.

- **Tennis Ball Squeeze:** Keep a tennis ball or other type of ball, soft or hard, at your desk, in the car, or around the house. Squeeze at least 10 times a day (more if you want). This improves that all-important vise-grip strength, and remember that as we age, grip strength is an all-important marker for preventing disability and frailty.

◆ THERAPY PUTTY ◆

If squeezing a tennis ball seems like not much fun, try Therapy Putty (you can find it at multiple online retailers, including Amazon). It's bright and colorful and comes in a variety of strengths. The medium is more challenging than you might think, but it'll take you back to your Silly Putty days, plus it's a terrific stress reducer—squeezing it also reduces your blood pressure.

- **Stand Up/Sit Down:** This is one you can do anywhere, as many times as you want. Simply get up from your chair (do not use a chair with wheels) without using your arms to push you up. Do not lean forward to get momentum; the object is to use your leg muscles. Then sit slowly all the way back down into the chair, focusing on your quads, the muscles at the fronts of your thighs. As your quad muscles get stronger, go down until you're almost but not quite sitting, and then come back up. This is a good exercise to do while you're talking on the phone. Start off with 3 sets of 10, two to four times a week.
- **Wall Sit:** If your legs are weak or the Stand Up/Sit Down exercise is hard on your knees, start off with a Wall Sit instead. Place your butt, back, and shoulders flat against the wall, with your feet about hip-distance apart about 1.5 feet away from the wall. Slide your back down the wall so your knees are bending. Go as low as you can go to start (the goal is to form a 90-degree angle with your bent knees—if you do it right, your body should look like it's sitting in an invisible chair). Hold this for a count of 5, then slide back up the wall. Repeat with your feet straight ahead, and again with your toes facing inward. As you get stronger, slide farther down the wall until your legs are at a 90-degree angle and you are holding for a count of 10. Start off with 2 sets of 5, two to four times a week.

Step Away from the Television Set

A 2008 Australian study of more than four thousand physically active adults showed that TV viewing time was positively associated with the risk of developing metabolic syndrome. In other words, even people who exercise need to cut down on the time they spend sitting still. The best advice is to cut down on TV time and computer time and get moving—walking, gardening, even doing household chores (you can always keep the TV on in the background, which is what my wife does). A pro football player told *Sports Illustrated* a few years ago that he watched hours and hours of TV—but he also did hundreds of push-ups and sit-ups while watching. That's what kept him from becoming an out-of-shape couch potato. If you don't want to give up your TV time, move while you watch. Take out that tennis ball and squeeze away. Sit on a stationary bike and pedal to your heart's content. Do your isometric exercises. Just keep moving—your body will thank you for it.

How much exercise is enough? Here's what I say: Aim for at least 30 minutes of moderate-intensity exercise—in addition to your customary activities—on most if not all days of the week (the more the better), then gradually build up to 1 hour a day. Moderate intensity is defined as burning 4 to 7 calories per minute, or any activity as intense as a brisk walk, mowing the lawn, dancing, swimming, or bicycling on level terrain. Also, aim for at least two days a week of strength-training exercises (such as stairs, Stand Up/Sit Down). If you haven't been active for a while, begin with short amounts of light-intensity activity and gradually increase the duration and intensity until you reach your goal. Don't have an hour to spare? How about ten minutes? You can make it easier to do by breaking up your exercise sessions into smaller sessions; you don't have to work out for sixty minutes all at one time. Instead you can try for four 15-minute sessions, six 10-minute sessions, two 30-minute sessions—whatever works best for you.

Week 3: Watch Your Waistline Daily Exercise Planner

The chart below is an example of how you can add waist-watching exercises to your SuperHealth program. Don't feel guilty if you eliminate one day of exercise. Everyone deserves a day of rest.

	Exercise	Set Reminders
Day 1	Walk	15 minutes
	Power Stairs	5 minutes
	Heel to Fanny	3 sets of 10
	Isometric Curl	10 times with both arms
	Isometric Extension	10 times with both arms
	Ball Squeeze	10 times
Day 2	Walk	15 minutes
	Heel to Fanny	3 sets of 10
	Sit-up/Crunch	3 sets of 10
	Isometric Curl	10 times with both arms
	Isometric Extension	10 times with both arms
Day 3	Walk	15 minutes
	Power Stairs	5 minutes
	Ball Squeeze	10 times
	Stand Up/Sit Down/Wall Sit	Unlimited times
Day 4	Walk	15 minutes
	Heel to Fanny	3 sets of 10
	Sit-up/Crunch	3 sets of 10
	Isometric Curl	10 times with both arms
	Isometric Extension	10 times with both arms
	Ball Squeeze	10 times
	Stand Up/Sit Down/Wall Sit	Unlimited times
Day 5	Walk	15 minutes
	Power Stairs	5 minutes
	Isometric Curl	10 times with both arms
	Isometric Extension	10 times with both arms
	Ball Squeeze	10 times
Day 6	Walk	15 minutes
	Heel to Fanny	3 sets of 10

(continued)

	Exercise	Set Reminders
Day 6 (*cont.*)	Sit-up/Crunch	3 sets of 10
	Ball Squeeze	10 times
	Stand Up/Sit Down/Wall Sit	Unlimited times
Day 7	Walk	15 minutes
	Power Stairs	5 minutes
	Isometric Curl	10 times with both arms
	Isometric Extension	10 times with both arms

WAIST WATCHING, BURNING CALORIES, AND BLOOD SUGAR

Blood sugar is like gasoline to an engine: No matter how good-looking the chassis, the car is not going anywhere without fuel. And if you want that engine to perform efficiently and to its maximum capacity, you'll choose the highest-quality, most appropriate fuel available.

If only we did the same when fueling our bodies. We get most of our energy from carbohydrates, which produce glucose, which becomes our blood sugar. The glucose circulates throughout the body and is used for energy. In an ideal world we'd eat just the right amount of carbohydrates to produce the energy we need. In fact, the body has a system of checks and balances between two hormones—insulin and glucagon—to help keep blood sugar levels on an even keel. But our bodies were designed to deal with whole, unprocessed foods found in nature (think SuperFoods); they weren't designed to cope with the bombardment of the highly processed, sugar-filled, trans-fat-laden, sodium-saturated goodies—or is it baddies?—of our modern world.

Here's why blood sugar levels are so important: The carbohydrates you consume get digested and turned into glucose. When glucose levels rise, insulin, produced in the pancreas, begins to do its job, which is to escort glucose into the liver and muscles, where it's turned into glycogen (the storage form of glucose). If there's more glucose than there is cell storage space, the excess is converted into fat, which can build up around our vital organs and cause many of the problems discussed above.

Once the glucose is in the cells, it's locked in place as glycogen. We need the second hormone, glucagon (also produced in the pancreas), to convert glycogen back to glucose so that it can be used for fuel.

When you eat a balanced diet, the counteraction of the two hormones works to keep your fasting blood sugar level in the normal range, which is between 70 and 100 milligrams of glucose per deciliter of blood (see page 341 to find out how to get your blood levels tested).

YOU CAN HELP CONTROL YOUR BLOOD SUGAR WITH FOOD AND EXERCISE

As you can see, blood sugar levels are extremely important to your health and longevity. High blood sugar levels can be a warning flag that you're aging faster than you should be. And unlike telltale signs like wrinkles and gray hair, your fasting blood sugar doesn't show up in the mirror. So don't be shy about asking your doctor to test your blood sugar, even if you're feeling fine. Regulating your blood sugar level is the most effective way of maintaining your fat-burning capacity. The good news is that blood sugar can be controlled largely by following the SuperHealth plan, adding fiber to your diet and incorporating exercise into your lifestyle.

- **Fiber and blood sugar:** We started off this week's SuperHealth plan with fruit and whole grains because of their dietary fiber contents. Recent research has shown that dietary fiber, especially whole grain bran, increases whole-body glucose disposal independent of changes in body weight, in both short- and long-term studies. Your body is continually trying to regulate the amount of sugar in your blood over a narrow range. Fiber helps to release the sugar more slowly into your blood. A glass of sugar water, for instance, will deposit that sugar into your system in a couple of minutes. So even when you're battling the bulge, dietary fiber comes to your rescue by helping to control blood sugar and insulin levels.

Don't Forget the Cinnamon

Cinnamon may not be a dietary fiber, but it sure acts like one. Cinnamon delays gastric emptying and slows the release of blood sugar. It slows down the speed at which food leaves your stomach, which in turn slows down the speed at which sugar enters your bloodstream. Cinnamon is a delicious companion to many of the foods in this chapter, including pumpkin, oatmeal, and cold cereal. You can also combine 1 cup of nonfat yogurt with 1 teaspoon of cinnamon and 1 to 2 teaspoons of honey, which you can serve as a dip for sliced fruit, as a dressing for fruit salad, or as a topper for whole grain pancakes, waffles, or granola.

- **Exercise and blood sugar:** At first glance it may seem puzzling what exercise has to do with blood sugar. The answer to this puzzle is, in part, muscle mass. Muscles store excess blood sugar (glucose) in the form of glycogen. As we get older, and/or as we get more sedentary, we lose muscle mass. That means we also lose some of our glucose storage capacity. When there's too much glucose in the blood, you have diabetes. As lean body mass (that is, muscle) increases, greater amounts of blood glucose are cleared from the blood. That is why any type of exercise that helps build muscle mass is part of a SuperHealth lifestyle.

Of course there are many more reasons to exercise than just controlling your blood sugar:

- **Exercise cuts the risk of heart disease.** By now just about everyone knows that exercise is good for the heart. But you may not know that it's good for more than preventing a heart attack—if you start regular physical exercise *after* you've had a heart attack, you have a much better chance of long-term survival and a better quality of life. The best news is that walking turns out to be a good way to cut the risk of heart disease—and it doesn't even have to be fast-paced. All you have to do is walk one hour a week. That works out to less than ten minutes a day! Of course I (and the U.S. Department of Health and Human Services) recommend more than that, but if you're a couch potato now, you can certainly find ten minutes a day for a walk around the neighborhood, and you can keep building from there.
- **Exercise lowers triglyceride levels.** There is evidence that aerobic exercise performed several hours before a fatty meal reduces the amount of postprandial (after-meal) triglycerides, a type of fat that contributes to atherosclerosis. One study had participants exercising for ninety minutes on the treadmill either thirty minutes before or ninety minutes after a meal of chocolate ice cream with whipped cream (sounds like my kind of study). The premeal exercise caused a 49 percent decrease and the postmeal exercise caused a 52 percent decrease. Because the heart expended more effort in the postmeal effort, the researchers recommended that anyone with a cardiac disorder exercise before a meal rather than after.
- **Exercise lowers blood pressure.** Exercise is also important for another heart-related subject: blood pressure. At present more than 65 million Americans have high blood pressure, or hypertension. Hypertension is dangerous because it causes the heart to work extra-hard. The less your heart has to work, the less pressure is exerted on your arteries. The ideal blood pressure condition in a normal

healthy person is less than 120/80mm Hg. The higher your blood pressure is to begin with, the more dramatic the decrease with exercise will be. And since blood pressure tends to rise as you age, it's important to keep exercising as you get older.

- **Exercise cuts cancer risk.** There are still many unknowns about cancer, about why a particular cancer attacks a particular person, why people react to similar cancers in vastly different ways, why one person survives a treatment protocol and another does not. We are getting more and more answers every day, although there is still much to be learned. One thing we do know, even though we don't know exactly why, is that physical activity helps prevent cancer. The answer may have to do with obesity and weight gain, two factors that are related to the cause of several cancers. Exercise influences hormone levels, which may have an effect on cancer. Exercise speeds up the passage of digested foods through the colon, reducing the time the colon lining is in contact with possible cancer-causing chemicals. Whatever the reasons, study after study has proved by convincing evidence that it works.

- **Exercise benefits the brain.** If, after reading everything in this chapter so far, you're still not motivated to get yourself moving, consider this: Physical exercise decreases your chances of developing Alzheimer's disease or losing cognitive function. In fact, a five-year study out of Quebec suggests that the more you exercise, the greater the protective benefits for the brain. Those in the study who did not exercise were twice as likely to develop Alzheimer's disease as compared to those who exercised vigorously at least three times a week—but even those who exercised less still cut their risk significantly. Studies have shown that both men and women benefit from walking; it has been shown to be associated with reduced risk of dementia and better cognitive function. One study even showed that the cognitive benefits of physical activity such as walking were similar to being about three years younger and were associated with a 20 percent lower risk of cognitive impairment.

- **Exercise keeps us standing.** Exercise not only keeps arthritis and osteoporosis at bay; it also helps us guard against sarcopenia. Sarcopenia (from the Greek meaning "poverty of flesh") is degenerative loss of muscle mass and strength in mature adults. Just as you lose bone mass as you get older, you also lose muscle mass. One of the strongest causative factors of sarcopenia is reduced physical activity. In other words, use it or lose it. When you don't exercise, you accelerate the loss of muscle mass, which causes more difficulty and discomfort. So I urge you, no matter what stage or age you are at currently, keep moving. The best way to prevent sarcopenia is to do exercises that provide resistance against your muscles—isometrics, Stand Up/Sit Down (page 107), and lifting light weights, for instance, are all good for preventing sarcopenia.

Play On!

Some people do it to classical music. Some people do it to hip-hop. Some even do it to show tunes. No matter what the genre, everybody knows it's easier to exercise if there's music playing. But now there's evidence suggesting that working out to music can actually give your brain a boost. A group of cardiac rehabilitation patients were given a verbal fluency test before and after two separate sessions of exercising on a treadmill. In one of the sessions participants listened to Vivaldi's *The Four Seasons*. The improvement in verbal fluency test performance after listening to the music was more than twice that of the nonaccompanied session. Now we know that music is not only the food of love; it's the fuel of the brain!

- **Exercise keeps us sexy.** It's not only our muscle mass that decreases as we age. Testosterone levels in men decline as well (which actually contributes to loss of muscle mass), which leads to decreased sexual function, among other things. However, a recent study of 102 men ages forty to seventy-five showed that those who exercised the most (six hours a week) increased levels of both the hormone dihydrotestosterone (DHT), the most active form of testosterone, and the sex hormone binding globulin SHBG, which binds to testosterone in the blood and actually makes it less biologically available. Some scientists believe that the more free testosterone (DHT), the greater the risk of prostate cancer. However, exercise studies suggest just the opposite. Low levels of DHT are associated with decreased prostate cancer survival rates, and low SHBG is associated with an increase in insulin resistance and metabolic syndrome. But as this study shows, exercise increases the levels of both of these substances. This shows just how important exercise can be to all aspects of health. For the complete Week 3 Planner, see page 296.

◆ MEET MILTON MULDAWER ◆

Exerciser of the Month

Before Milton Muldawer's wife passed away in 2005, he was "more or less" a couch potato. He watched a lot of TV, did a lot of reading. Didn't do much of anything, in fact, that resembled physical activity. Even after he was diagnosed with diabetes, he was not motivated to get off the sofa.

But when his wife died, Muldawer realized he had to start taking care of himself. He started eating better. "I don't eat as well as I should," he says, "because I'm alone. I buy a lot of prepared meals from Costco and from the kosher market in the neighborhood. But I have fish several times a week—salmon, tilapia, rainbow trout. I get frozen vegetables like string beans, snap peas, and broccoli mix. And I have a big salad every day with lettuce, tomatoes, celery, cucumbers, and red and green peppers."

But what Muldawer does most these days is exercise. In the winter he walks around the mall, about a mile and a half twice a week (he was walking two miles, but recently he's slowed down a bit). He goes to exercise class twice a week, and he also works with a personal trainer who helps him work out on various body-strengthening machines another two days, working all the different muscle groups. That's six days a week of one kind of exercise or another. Not long ago the gym he attends voted him "exerciser of the month" for all his efforts. Not bad for a former couch potato.

"There are many days I just don't feel like going," says Muldawer. "I have to give myself a kick in the rear to get out the door. It would be so much easier just to stay home, sit in a chair, and read. But I always feel better after I exercise. And I've lost about sixteen pounds, so I don't want to stop now."

It's not always easy to maintain the weight loss. He's gained one or two pounds in the past few months and says he's just going to have to try a little bit harder. Because, he says, he enjoys it when people notice that he's lost weight and tell him how good he looks. "That's a great compliment," he says. "And I love to see their faces when I tell them I'm ninety-one years old."

6

Step 4: Control Inflammation

For your basics, see the SuperHealth Food Pyramid,
page 19 (for your bonus see below)

Week 4 SuperFoods:

Wild salmon
Skinless turkey breast
Garlic

Extra virgin olive oil
Oats

Fire, heat, is essential to life. It keeps us warm, it helps
regulate the immune system's ability to combat infection, and it makes certain foods more bioavailable to
our bodies. But our environment of toxins, with bad
fats and too much sugar, is like pouring gasoline on a
fire lit in a hearth—pretty soon it gets out of control
and burns the whole house down. That's what's happening to our bodies, but if we counteract that gasoline
by eating the right SuperFoods, exercising, getting a
good night's sleep, and reducing stress, we can reduce
the cause of almost all major illness: inflammation.

How does controlling inflammation help you live
longer? In trying to determine why we get sick, scientists recently have begun to believe that inflammation
may be at the heart (and lungs and brain and all other

body parts) of virtually all the diseases we suffer from, and that controlling inflammation may be one of the most potent tools we have for living longer, more disease-free lives.

In the simplest sense, inflammation occurs as an immune response when tissue has been injured or irritated or has become diseased. It is the first response of the immune system to any abnormal occurrence in the body. When foreign irritants invade the body, inflammation rushes in to the rescue, initiating the healing process for the tissue under attack. Our bodies use inflammation to repair damaged tissue and to kill pathogens such as bacteria and fungi. Inflammation is an essential part of the immune system's defense mechanism.

If we didn't have any inflammatory processes, we'd be dead in no time. Not only does inflammation allow us to deal with a multitude of living and nonliving substances that enter our bodies, but it is an essential component of our body's reparative mechanisms.

But ... inflammation is a double-edged sword. It can get out of hand. For example, if there is too much inflammation in a joint, instead of repairing that joint, it can cause diseases like rheumatoid arthritis or osteoarthritis. Inflammatory responses are present in all of our cells and play a role in their eventual breakdown. When it goes overboard, it is the precursor to most diseases, including cardiovascular disease, stroke, cancer, diabetes, Alzheimer's disease, macular degeneration, and cataracts, and it plays a central role in speeding up the aging process.

Chronic inflammation may be fueled by a broad range of lifestyle factors that promote the production of inflammatory chemicals, including smoking, stress, chronic sleep deprivation (less than seven hours a night), being overweight, lack of exercise, and—you guessed it—diet.

Fighting inflammation all starts, of course, with adding SuperFoods to your diet. All twenty-five Super-Foods will help you in that respect, but in this chapter we're going to concentrate on the five that are particularly effective in fighting inflammation: wild salmon, skinless turkey breast, garlic, extra virgin olive oil, and oats. You have been introduced to some of these foods previously, but now you'll find out how they can prevent you from burning up before you flame out.

Wild Salmon

Recommended amount: 3 to 4 ounces (1 deck of cards), two to four times a week.

Sidekicks: Alaskan/northern halibut, canned chunk light or albacore tuna, mackerel, herring, sardines, farmed trout, cod, shrimp, sea bass, oysters, and clams (farmed or wild)

While salmon is rich in protein, B vitamins, potassium, selenium, and other important minerals, it's the ample supply of omega-3 fatty acids that makes it so important as a health-promoting food. That's why wild salmon was introduced as one of the first SuperFoods for your SuperHealth plan—because the most important step you can take to prevent chronic inflammation is to have the right ratio of omega-3 fatty acids to omega-6 fatty acids. An added bonus of my favorite wild Alaskan salmon, sockeye, is that it is loaded with the carotenoids astaxanthin and zeaxanthin, phytonutrients found in foods that are essential for achieving and maintaining SuperHealth, which most likely add to its overall anti-inflammatory punch.

When we eat too many unhealthy fats and refined and processed foods, the crucial omega-6/omega-3 ratio gets out of whack. That kind of unbalanced diet assaults the immune system and encourages inflammation. A processed-foods diet is also lacking in naturally occurring antioxidants and phytonutrients, which help the body fight inflammation. You can reduce inflammation by emphasizing foods that decrease the body's production of inflammatory compounds, like the foods listed in this chapter (and all the other SuperFoods as well).

Skinless Turkey Breast

Recommended amount: 3 to 4 ounces (1 deck of cards), three to four times a week

Sidekick: skinless chicken breast

Skinless turkey breast is one of the leanest meat protein sources on the planet. That means it is very low in saturated fat. Too much saturated fat (and trans fat) overpromotes inflammation and therefore promotes disease. In addition to its low level of saturated fat, turkey has a rich array of healthy nutrients, including riboflavin, niacin, vitamins B_6 and B_{12}, iron, and—most important in relation to bringing inflammation into balance—selenium and zinc.

Selenium is vital in the utilization and function of glutathione and glutathione antioxidant-containing enzyme systems, which help detoxify the body. It is also an antioxidant that helps protect the body by neutralizing free radicals that harm cells. And it helps activate prostaglandins, hormone-like chemical messengers that are involved in a wide range of body functions, including helping to control the inflammatory process. People who live in selenium-poor regions of the world suffer from dramatically increased rates of cancer, infections, and inflammatory diseases. (Some soils are naturally poor in selenium, so foods grown in these soils are low in this important micromineral as well. For example, parts of the Pacific Northwest and parts of the Great Lakes region have selenium-deficient soil, as does the Linxian area of China.) Zinc is required for the development and activation of T lymphocytes, a kind of white blood cell that helps fight infection. So if you want to help lower inflammation, you might want to think about turkey weekly instead of yearly.

When buying turkey at a deli, ask for fresh roasted turkey meat if available. The turkey breast found in delis and supermarkets usually contains fillers as well as high amounts of fat and sodium. You can also use fresh ground turkey in place of ground beef for burgers, sauces, tacos, enchiladas, stir-fries, sandwiches, and casseroles (check the label for turkey that is 97 to 99 percent fat free). See pages 283 and 284 for some delicious turkey recipes.

What About Chicken?

While chicken is listed here as a sidekick, it's not on an equal footing with turkey breast. That's because skinless roasted chicken is higher in calories and saturated fat than roasted skinless white meat turkey. As with turkey, stick with the white meat breast of the chicken for maximum health benefits.

Garlic

Recommended amount: to taste three or more times a week; garlic powder is fine, but if you want to maximize the benefits, go with fresh.

Sidekicks: scallions, shallots, leeks, onions

Garlic, which we met in Chapter 4 as a detoxifier, is a major player in many cuisines around the world. As far back as 2600 B.C. garlic was known for its medicinal properties. Egyptians used garlic to enhance the strength and endurance of the slaves who built the pyramids. Garlic is a potent anti-inflammatory agent. It contains nearly one hundred nutrients that, working together, give it effective antioxidant and anti-inflammatory abilities.

Garlic is available in supplement form, but I believe that fresh garlic is a much better choice, as it provides more health benefits than the powdered form. When shopping for garlic, look for cloves that are plump and without blemishes—don't buy cloves that are soft, shriveled, or moldy, or that have begun to sprout. Just one clove or even half a clove of finely minced raw garlic in dressings, dips, soups, stews, and pasta sauce adds great flavor without overpowering the dish. But if you're a garlic lover like I am, use as much as you like.

Spice It Up to Turn Down the Heat

Apparently Mother Nature is nurturing us well by providing us with condiments that not only make our food tastier but make it healthier as well. Many spices are rich in antioxidants, which work by gobbling up free radicals that can lead to chronic inflammation. Spices that have been found to have anti-inflammatory properties should be used liberally to taste whenever possible—at least one meal a day. Here are a few of them:

- **Cinnamon:** A 2006 study published in the *Federation of American Societies for Experimental Biology Journal* showed that cinnamon, like insulin, increases the amount of three critically important proteins involved in the body's insulin signaling, glucose transport, and inflammatory response. One of the researchers for this study, Dr. Richard Anderson of the U.S. Department of Agriculture, told *Medical News Today* that "[a]s an anti-inflammatory agent, cinnamon may be useful in preventing or mitigating arthritis as well as cardiovascular disease." And as scientists increasingly understand the relationship between inflammation and insulin function in Alzheimer's disease, cinnamon's ability to block inflammation and enhance insulin function may make it useful in combating that disease as well.

- **Ginger:** Ginger has been used as both a spice and an herbal medicine for thousands of years. It is known to prevent and relieve nausea, indigestion, pain, and inflammation, and is widely used to reduce arthritic symptoms. Ginger has been shown to contain powerful anti-inflammatory properties. Ginger also suppresses the production of a number of pro-inflammatory cytokines (proteins that facilitate communication among immune system cells) and reduces the pain of arthritis for many patients. Fresh ginger is available in the pro-

(*continued*)

duce section of most grocery stores, in crystallized form, and powdered. It's also used in tea and other beverages (which is why your mother always gave you ginger ale to calm an upset stomach).

- **Turmeric:** Most of the world's supply of turmeric, a member of the same family of plants as ginger, comes from India, where it is widely used as the ingredient that gives curry its unique flavor and yellow color. Like ginger, turmeric is known to have anti-inflammatory properties and has been used to reduce the pain and inflammation of arthritis. And like cinnamon, curcumin (the antioxidant that gives turmeric its yellow hue) is also being studied for its possible use in the treatment and prevention of Alzheimer's disease. It is not known if anti-inflammatory approaches will cure Alzheimer's, but it appears likely that they can help slow the progression or delay the onset of this devastating disorder. You can take turmeric in the form of a supplement in Jarrow Formula's Circumin 95, 500 milligrams once or twice a day (www.jarrow.com), or the SuperFoods Spice supplement.

  Other anti-inflammatory spices include black pepper, basil, rosemary, thyme, and oregano. Use liberally—they may add years to your life.

Extra Virgin Olive Oil (EVOO)

Recommended amount: 1 to 2 tablespoons most days
Sidekick: canola oil

One of the best ways to reduce inflammation is by emphasizing healthful fats (for example, omega-3 fatty acids and monounsaturated fats) that decrease the body's production of inflammatory compounds, fight harmful free radicals, and boost the immune system. Extra virgin olive oil has what it takes to do the job. A 2005 study revealed that a compound in extra virgin olive oil called oleocanthal prevents the production of pro-inflammatory COX-1 and COX-2 enzymes—the same way nonsteroidal anti-inflammatory drugs (NSAIDs), such as ibuprofen and aspirin, work. Luckily, however, olive oil does not damage the stomach or promote the development of peptic ulcers, as do aspirin and other anti-inflammatory drugs.

Oats

Recommended amount: 10 grams of whole grain fiber a day as part of your goal of 32 grams of dietary fiber per day for women and 45 grams of fiber a day for men (see the chart on page 91)

Sidekicks: wheat germ, ground flaxseed, brown rice, barley, wheat, buckwheat, rye, millet, bulgar wheat, amaranth, quinoa, triticale, kamut, yellow corn, wild rice, spelt

We already know that fiber is good for your heart because it helps lower cholesterol. Oats, for instance, contain soluble fiber that binds with and helps remove some of the cholesterol that can clog your arteries and lead to heart disease. However, recent studies have shown that a high fiber intake (at least 30 grams a day) significantly reduces inflammation levels. C-reactive protein (CRP), produced by the liver, is a protein that rises when there is bodywide (systemic) inflammation. CRP is used mainly as a marker of inflammation—the higher the number, the higher your risk for cardiovascular events such as heart attack and stroke. A CRP level below 1 mg/L (milligrams per liter) is best; 1 to 3 mg/L indicates a moderate risk of inflammation; and anything above 3 mg/L is a high risk.

Researchers from the Medical University of South Carolina put a group of volunteers on a high-fiber diet, and what they found was that overall their levels of CRP decreased by 13.7 percent, which suggests a lowered risk for multiple chronic diseases, such as macular degeneration and cardiovascular disease.

Absolute musts: If there's only one food for controlling inflammation you add this week, my recommendation is 2 to 4 servings of wild salmon or sidekicks.

Week 4: Control Inflammation Daily Planner

The chart below is an example of how you can add inflammation-fighting foods to your SuperHealth program. It shows you how to get inflammation-controlling foods into your diet—but it doesn't mean these are the only foods you should eat for the week. They are just suggestions; feel free to mix and match foods and days to your heart's content (and health).

	Food Suggestion	**Daily Servings**
Day 1	Wild salmon	3–4 ounces (1 deck of cards)
	Flaxseed	2 tablespoons ground (1 shot glass)
	Garlic	To taste
	EVOO	2 tablespoons (1 shot glass)
	Spices	To taste
Day 2	Skinless turkey breast	3–4 ounces (1 deck of cards)
	Brown rice	½ cup (½ baseball)
	Garlic	To taste
	EVOO	2 tablespoons (1 shot glass)
	Spices	To taste
Day 3	Alaskan halibut	3–4 ounces (1 deck of cards)
	Quinoa	½ cup (½ baseball)
	Garlic	To taste
	EVOO	2 tablespoons (1 shot glass)
	Spices	To taste
Day 4	Skinless turkey breast	3–4 ounces (1 deck of cards)
	Barley	½ cup (½ baseball)
	Onion	¼ medium (¼ baseball)
	EVOO	2 tablespoons (1 shot glass)
	Spices	To taste
Day 5	Brown rice	½ cup (½ baseball)
	Leeks (raw or cooked)	½ cup (½ baseball) raw or cooked
	Yellow corn	½ cup (½ baseball)
	EVOO	2 tablespoons (1 shot glass)
	Spices	To taste

	Food Suggestion	Daily Servings
Day 6	Canned chunk light tuna	3–4 ounces (1 deck of cards)
	Whole grain bread	2 slices
	Scallions	½ cup (½ baseball)
	EVOO	2 tablespoons (1 shot glass)
	Spices	To taste
Day 7	Skinless turkey breast	3–4 ounces (1 deck of cards)
	Wild rice	½ cup (½ baseball)
	Garlic	To taste
	EVOO	2 tablespoons (1 shot glass)
	Spices	To taste

SHAKE YOUR GROOVE THING: EXERCISE AND INFLAMMATION

You might think that one way to live longer would be to just sit still and let your body do what it does. What harm (other than random natural disasters or airplanes falling from the sky) can come to you sitting in your easy chair? Plenty, it seems. It turns out that human beings were not built to be lazy.

Studies have shown over and over again that regular exercise helps you live longer, and scientists now believe that one of the reasons is that exercise reduces inflammation. When lack of physical activity is reported, higher levels of inflammatory markers associated with higher coronary heart disease risk are discovered. To show how dramatic results can be, one study put participants on a twelve-week aerobic and resistance training program and measured their CRP levels (an indication of inflammation) before and after. Half the group was between the ages of eighteen and thirty-five, and half the group was sixty-five and older. At the end of the twelve weeks, there was an average of a 58 percent decrease in CRP for both age groups.

Exercise is especially relevant as we get older and

possibly begin to suffer from loss of muscle mass and sarcopenia—the age-related loss of skeletal muscle mass and strength. SuperHealth requires muscle. It's apparent in my own practice that when my older patients start having trouble standing up when called into the exam room, the walker and further decline are just around the corner.

There are several theories about the genesis of sarcopenia, one of which is that low-grade inflammation is an important contributor to the process. It has been established that muscle tissue is responsive to a number of proinflammatory chemicals. Several studies have shown that decreased physical activity with aging appears to be the key factor involved in producing sarcopenia—which means that if you want to be able to move around as you get older, you've got to lower your levels of inflammation, and one great way to do that is to keep moving around.

That means continuing and increasing the exercise portion of the SuperHealth program you started in Week 3:

- **Walk the walk:** Increase your walking time to at least 20 minutes, four to five days a week. If you counted your steps last week via your pedometer, increase your amount by 500 steps for this week. So if you started last week with 3,500 steps each day, your goal for this week is 4,000 steps each day.
- **Dr. Steve's Power Stairs Workout:** Increase the number of times you walk up and down the stairs in your home or office. If you were doing 5 minutes last week, try for two to four days of 7 minutes each day this week and increase the speed at which you walk.
- **Heel to Fanny:** Stand on stairs or an elevated area (this can be done on a flat surface as well) and hold on to the railing or the wall keeping your knees together. The left leg remains straight. With your right leg beginning in a straight position, bring your right heel to your fanny. You may not be able to

touch your fanny, but take it as far as you can go and hold it there for 3 seconds, then let it down slowly. Increase to 3 sets of 15 with each leg three to four days a week. This builds strength in the hamstrings, those big muscles in the back of the thigh.

- **Sit-up/Crunch:** Lie on your back with your knees bent and your feet flat on the floor in front of you. Lie on an exercise mat or carpet rather than a hard floor to prevent back strain. Your feet should be as wide apart as your hips. Place your arms crossed on your chest and keep your chin pointing upward. Curl up and forward so that your head, neck, and shoulder blades lift off the floor. Pause for a count of one, then slowly lower your shoulder blades, neck, and head to starting position. Increase to three sets of 20, three days a week.

- **Isometric Curl:** Hold on to the back of the steering wheel (while at a stop sign or signal) at the five o'clock and seven o'clock positions with your palms facing toward you and your arms bent. This can also be done by grabbing the edge of a desk or table, palms facing up, elbows at your sides, shoulders down. The idea is to attempt to bring your hands up toward your shoulders (you won't actually be able to do it—the point is to get the resistance). Hold the position for 10 to 20 seconds and repeat 15 times using both arms. This helps to tone the biceps and the front part of the shoulder muscles. For maximum benefit, vary the amount of arm bend slightly for each rep, as this strengthens the muscle at varying degrees of use. Make sure to keep your shoulders down and back. Do this two to four days a week.

- **Isometric Extension:** Again, this is a nonmovement form of strengthening. This time you're pushing against the steering wheel, desk, or any other immobile surface, with the heel of your hand and your fingers pointing down. Try to extend or straighten your arms, using your body weight to resist. Hold the position for 10 to 20 seconds and repeat 15 times using both arms. This helps to tone the triceps (back of the arm). Do this two to four days a week.

- **Tennis Ball Squeeze:** Keep a tennis ball or other type of ball, soft or hard, at your desk, in the car, or around the house. Squeeze at least 20 times a day (more if you want). Squeezing the ball and holding it for a count of 20 can actually help lower your blood pressure. It's a good one to do while you're on the phone during a stressful conversation—stress is a major source of inflammation.

- **Stand Up/Sit Down:** This is one you can do anywhere, as many times as you want. Simply get up from your chair (do not use a chair with wheels) without using your arms to push you up. Do not lean forward to get momentum; the object is to use your leg muscles. Then sit slowly all the way back down into the chair, focusing on your quads, the muscles at the fronts of your thighs. As your quad muscles get stronger, go down until you're almost but not quite sitting, and then come back up. This is another good exercise to do while you're talking on the phone. This week, do 3 sets of 15, two to four times.

- **Wall Sit:** If your legs are weak or the Stand Up/Sit Down exercise is hard on your knees, start off with a Wall Sit instead. Place your butt, back, and shoulders flat against the wall, with your feet about hip-distance apart about 1.5 feet away from the wall. Slide your back down the wall so your knees are bending. Go as low as you can go to start (the goal is to form a 90-degree angle with your bent knees—if you do it right, your body should look like it's sitting in an invisible chair). Hold this for a count of 5, then slide back up the wall. Repeat with your feet straight ahead, and again with your toes facing inward. As you get stronger, slide farther down the wall until your legs are at a 90-degree angle and you are holding for a count of 10. This week, do 3 sets of 15, two to four times.

Most of the exercises above are actually part of resistance (strength) training, perhaps the most essential tool you can find for extending your SuperHealth potential. Resistance training is a term for exercises that build and maintain muscles by harnessing resistance, meaning an opposing force that muscles strain against. That can mean anything from working an old-fashioned can opener, carrying out the garbage, digging a hole in the garden, shoveling dirt, walking up or down stairs or hills, to lifting, doing pull-ups, push-ups, and chin-ups. Resistance can be supplied by your body, free weights (dumbbells), weighted cuffs (wrist or ankle weights), elastic bands, or specialized weight-training machines.

It's about more than just building body strength—it enhances your ability to lead an active, independent life, and to enjoy your friends and family, your pets, and your relationships long after maturity begins to rear its sometimes ugly head. Resistance training reduces the risk factors associated with coronary heart disease, type 2 diabetes, and colon cancer; it also helps prevent osteoporosis, promotes weight loss and maintenance, improves balance (reducing your chances of falling as you age), and promotes general well-being. It has been recognized in both scientific and medical communities that muscular strength is a fundamental physical trait necessary for health, functional ability, and enhanced quality of life.

No matter what kind of resistance you use, putting more than the usual amount of load on your muscles makes them strong. And because muscles are attached to bones, this will help make the bones stronger as well—not to mention what it does for your posture and appearance.

This week, try these three additional resistance exercises:

- **Steering Wheel Squeeze:** While parked or at a red light, grip the steering wheel so that your hands are horizontally across from each other (at the three o'clock and nine o'clock positions). Your elbows are out and your arms should be forming a "C" shape. Try to push your hands together against the steering wheel—imagine that you're trying to close the "C" shape of your arms into an "O" shape. Hold this for 5 to 10 seconds, then let go. Repeat 10 times. This is great for building the forearms, biceps, and shoulder muscles. You can try it outside the car too: Grab either side of the back of a chair and try to push your arms from a "C" into an "O." Do this two to four days a week.

- **Bicep Curl:** Stand with your feet about hip-width apart as you hold a light weight in each hand in front of the thighs. If you are just beginning, choose a weight that allows you to easily do three sets of ten curls (you can also use cans of soup or vegetables if you don't have weights). Your grip should be underhand (palms facing upward). Squeeze your biceps and bend your arms, curling the weights up toward your shoulders. Keep your elbows stationary and at the sides of your body and bring the weights only as high as you can without moving your elbows. Slowly lower the weights, keeping a slight bend in the elbows at the bottom (don't lock the joints; try to keep tension on the muscle). Repeat for 3 sets of 10 reps, two to three times a week.

- **Tricep Extension:** From a standing position with your feet about hip-width apart, hold a light weight (or can) in your right hand. Bend forward so that your upper torso is perpendicular to the floor, keeping your right arm straight at your side. Bend and raise your elbow up toward the ceiling until your arm is at a right angle at your side, then extend your arm backward until it's straight. Hold and lower slowly. Repeat for 3 sets of 10, then repeat with your left arm. Do this two to four days a week.

Week 4: Control Inflammation Daily Exercise Planner

	Exercise	Set Reminders
Day 1	Walk	20 minutes
	Power Stairs	7 minutes
	Heel to Fanny	3 sets of 15
	Isometric Curl	15 times with both arms
	Isometric Extension	15 times with both arms
	Ball Squeeze	20 times
	Steering Wheel Squeeze	10 times
Day 2	Walk	20 minutes
	Heel to Fanny	3 sets of 15
	Sit-up/Crunch	3 sets of 20
	Isometric Curl	15 times with both arms
	Isometric Extension	15 times with both arms
	Bicep Curl	3 sets of 10
	Tricep Extension	3 sets of 10
Day 3	Walk	20 minutes
	Power Stairs	7 minutes
	Ball Squeeze	20 times
	Stand Up/Sit Down/Wall Sit	3 sets of 15
	Steering Wheel Squeeze	10 times
Day 4	Walk	20 minutes
	Heel to Fanny	3 sets of 15
	Sit-up/Crunch	3 sets of 20
	Isometric Curl	15 times with both arms
	Isometric Extension	15 times with both arms
	Ball Squeeze	20 times
	Stand Up/Sit Down/Wall Sit	3 sets of 15
Day 5	Walk	20 minutes
	Power Stairs	7 minutes
	Isometric Curl	15 times with both arms
	Isometric Extension	15 times with both arms
	Ball Squeeze	20 times
	Bicep Curl	3 sets of 10
	Tricep Extension	3 sets of 10
Day 6	Walk	20 minutes
	Heel to Fanny	3 sets of 15

(continued)

	Exercise	**Set Reminders**
Day 6 (*cont.*)	Sit-up/Crunch	3 sets of 20
	Ball Squeeze	20 times
	Stand Up/Sit Down/Wall Sit	3 sets of 15
	Steering Wheel Squeeze	10 times
Day 7	Walk	20 minutes
	Power Stairs	7 minutes
	Isometric Curl	15 times with both arms
	Isometric Extension	20 times with both arms
	Bicep Curl	3 sets of 10
	Tricep Extension	3 sets of 10

THE INFLAMMATION CHALLENGE: MAKING LIFESTYLE CHANGES TO REDUCE INFLAMMATION

While some factors associated with inflammation, such as aging, can't be altered, embracing a healthy lifestyle—including a SuperHealth diet and exercise program, as well as getting more sleep and reducing stress levels—can dramatically decrease inflammation levels.

SLEEP, INFLAMMATION, AND THE IMMUNE SYSTEM

Imagine there was one thing you could do to lose weight, balance your hormones, get your appetite under control, help prevent heart disease, cancer, and arthritis (just to name a few), and in order to do it, you didn't have to move a muscle. You just have to lie flat on your back, your side, or your stomach, on a nice fluffy mattress, and drift off into dreamland. You just have to get enough sleep.

If you picture the SuperHealth program as a giant wheel with each of its six steps as spokes, at its very center you will find sleep. Sleep is the hub of SuperHealth. If you do everything else right—watch your diet, get in some exercise, practice stress-reducing behaviors—and then stay up late into the night to finish that last bit of work or watch late-night TV or play one last game on the computer, you're undermining all your positive efforts. The miraculous human body can adapt to a huge variety of lifestyle choices, but you can't adapt to lack of sleep.

How Much Is Enough and What Happens if You Don't Get Enough?

What happens when you stay up or get very little sleep for two nights to study for an exam or to complete a project on deadline? Or when you come back from a fun-filled party-hardy vacation? Usually what happens is that you get sick. Coincidence? No. This is something we've all experienced when under stress and pressing deadlines. You're working long hours, getting less sleep than usual, and next thing you know, you're flat on your back with a cold or the flu.

Studies have shown that even a modest loss of sleep (anything less than seven hours) for a single night increases inflammation. A 2005 UCLA research team conducted blood and DNA analyses of thirty healthy adults drawn during the day after partial-night sleep deprivation. The results showed that the immune system produced significantly greater amounts of two disease-fighting proteins after a night of sleep loss (which would be good if you actually had a disease—but when induced by sleep loss it paradoxically increases inflammation) compared with amounts found after a night of uninterrupted sleep.

What's even more interesting is that there's a delicate balancing act at work here, because the immune system has a role in regulating sleep.

When you're sleeping your body creates more anti-inflammatory cytokines, which means you have a better chance of fighting off infection. The less sleep you get, the fewer of these cytokines are produced, and the greater your chances of getting sick. Once you do get sick, the immune system kicks in to increase production of cytokines like interleukin-1 (IL-1), which is not only a powerful fighter against bacteria; it also acts as a sedative to help you get the sleep you need (when IL-1 is injected into animal brains, the animals fall asleep). So there is a cyclical interaction between the immune system and sleep: Sleep promotes the immune system and the immune system promotes sleep.

If You're Having Trouble Sleeping

If you are having an occasional problem sleeping, try some of these tips and see if they do the job:

- Go to bed at night and get up in the morning at the same time daily, even on weekends and holidays. Establish a routine and avoid variation as much as possible.
- Make your bed the place for sleep and sex. If you read in bed, read something relaxing—something that doesn't raise your pulse rate. Same for watching television. And turn off the computer at least one hour before you go to bed.
- Save your problems for the light of day. For couples bedtime is not the time to discuss your issues. Set aside a special time during the day for this activity so that you have time to relax and cool off before you try to get your nightly zzz's.
- Take turns massaging your partner—trade off every night. One night you rub your partner's back, the next night your partner rubs yours. It doesn't have to be a full-fledged deep-tissue massage; even just a gentle hand or foot rub can be a helpful bedtime ritual.
- Have dinner and drinks no later than three hours before bedtime. Caffeine can stay in your body for eight to twelve hours. Alcohol may help you get to sleep, but it keeps you in the lighter stages of sleep and you probably will wake up in the middle of the night when the sedating effects have worn off.
- Exercise no later than four hours before bedtime.

Studies show that exercise at night delays the release of melatonin that helps you fall asleep.

- Take a hot bath before bedtime. It does more than help you relax: When you get out of the tub, your body temperature drops in a way that mimics what happens as you fall asleep.

- If you take a nap during the day, keep it short and do it early in the day (before 3:00 p.m.). A power nap of fifteen to twenty minutes surprisingly can do wonders. Full sleep cycles, including settling the body and mind for sleep, going deeply to sleep, and the final dreaming stage, apparently recur during a night's sleep in 90- to 120-minute cycles. Power naps take advantage of the first two stages—relaxation and refreshing light sleep. But don't sleep longer than about twenty minutes or you'll wake up after the body has gone into deep sleep, which can leave you feeling fuzzy and still tired. After you do wake up, take a minute to reorient yourself by taking a few deep breaths and stretching to ease yourself back into your day.

Getting the Flu Vaccine? Get a Good Night's Sleep

Just when you think lack of sleep can't have one more consequence, up pops another one. A 2002 study from the University of Chicago showed that chronic sleep loss can impair the body's ability to develop antibodies. When sleep-deprived volunteers were given the flu vaccine, they built up less than half the amount of antibodies as volunteers who were well rested. So if you want to be sure you're getting full protection from any kind of vaccine, be sure you get enough sleep for several nights before you get immunized.

- Get out in the sun. Daylight is key to regulating sleep patterns. Try to get natural sunlight for at least thirty minutes each day. One thing I do myself is never put on sunglasses before 8:00 a.m. or after 4:00 p.m. Our bodies need exposure to sunlight to stay healthy. Light is processed by the eyes and then relayed as a chemical message to the brain, which in turn promotes melatonin production. Blind women, for instance, are at greater risk for breast cancer because their melatonin production is not as good. And melatonin helps you sleep at night. Blocking out all UVA, UVB, and blue light all the time is not best for your health.

- Install a red night-light in your hall or bathroom. Turning on the light when you go to the bathroom at night stops all melatonin production and you start all over again when you get back in bed and and try to go back to sleep. If you do need a light (you don't want to fall on the way there or back), it's better to have a low-voltage red night-light in the hallway or bathroom near the floor.

- If you can't sleep, get up. If you're still awake after twenty minutes, engage in a relaxing activity like stretching, reading, or listening to music until you feel sleepy.

Mom's Best Nighttime Trick

To help you fall asleep, try progressive muscle relaxation: Systematically relax each part of the body until the entire body is relaxed. Lie down in bed on your back and take slow, deep breaths. Starting with your toes, relax up to the top of your head, concentrating on one body part at a time. Make your body parts feel heavy; feel them relax. My mom taught me this just before I went off to college, and it has worked for me since 1963.

How Much Sleep Do We Need?

It's ironic that as children we are constantly fighting to stay awake as long as possible ("But Mommy, I'm not tired!" says Junior even as his eyes are involuntarily closing), while as adults we're constantly wishing we had more time to sleep. If you never had to get up to the alarm, just how much time would you sleep? Researchers have found that when adults are given an unlimited opportunity to sleep, they're down for an average of eight to eight and a half hours a night, and there is also another sleep period, twenty minutes to one hour, that occurs twelve hours after the midpoint of the long nighttime sleep period. Newborns sleep between sixteen and eighteen hours a day, while toddlers sleep between eight and ten hours. School-age children and adolescents need at least nine hours of sleep; studies have shown that kids between eleven and eighteen who get that amount of sleep consistently get better grades. The problem is that most teenagers get only about 6.9 to 7.5 hours of sleep a night. Typically teens want to go to bed later in the evening and sleep later in the morning. However, like adults who have to punch a clock, they have early-morning school starts, which is why they usually don't get enough sleep.

Over the years there have been many studies about what happens to people when they are deprived of a full night's sleep (or several nights' sleep), but far less research has been done on what is called partial sleep deprivation, or sleep debt, which is when you get less than seven hours of sleep a night for several consecutive nights. What studies have shown is that when you go into sleep debt your performance of daily tasks begins to suffer. You begin to have behavioral lapses, or so-called microsleeps, in which you doze off for as little as five to ten seconds or fall into a full-blown sleep attack from which you have trouble being aroused. In one study participants had either four or six hours of sleep a night for a two-week period. After fourteen days their behavioral lapses were the same as if they had been totally deprived of sleep for up to three days. It's clear that when healthy adults get less than seven hours of sleep a night the result is lapses of attention and performance that get progressively worse as the number of days in sleep debt increase.

In one study that followed more than 21,000 twins for over twenty-two years, researchers found that when people slept less than seven hours a night or more than eight hours a night, they had an increased risk of death. There was a 21 percent increase in risk of death for women who got shorter amounts of sleep and a 26 percent increase for men. These observations have been reported in a number of additional smaller studies; in summary they show a U-shaped relationship between sleep duration and all causes of mortality, suggesting that there is an optimal amount of sleep for healthy living. Sleep deprivation has been shown in any number of studies to be associated with a variety of health hazards:

- **Sleep and cardiac disease:** A 2003 study published in the *Journal of the American Medical Association* revealed that women who slept less than seven hours a night were found to have an increased risk of coronary events when compared to those who had eight hours a night. The risk was increased threefold for subjects who slept less than five hours at least twice a week. There may be a number of reasons for this. One possible cause is that people who chronically do not get enough sleep have higher blood levels of C-reactive protein, a sign that plaque is likely being formed in the arteries. Another possible reason is that when you enter the deep-sleep phases, your heart rate slows and your blood pressure drops by about 10 percent. Apparently this drop in blood pressure is important for your cardiovascular health. If you don't get enough sleep, and this dip in blood pressure does not occur, you are more likely to experience chest pain, an irregular heartbeat, a heart attack, or congestive heart failure in which fluid builds up in the body because the heart is not pumping sufficiently. For reasons not yet understood, in general African Americans do not have as much of a dip in blood pressure during sleep and are therefore at higher risk for cardiovascular disease. Sleep deprivation can also trigger the production of stress hormones such as adrenaline and cortisol, which can also inhibit the drop in blood pressure.

Mom Was Right Again

If you're going to have a heart attack or a stroke, you're more likely to have it in the morning, between 6 a.m. and noon, and particularly in the first hour after waking. There is a 49 percent increased risk in all types of stroke during this time of day. This may be due to the fact that blood pressure rises in the morning, stress hormones kick in as you rise and get ready for the hectic day ahead, and/or because platelets are "stickier" at this time of day and more likely to form blood clots.

My mother always advised us to drink an 8-ounce glass of water as soon as we got up in the morning. I always remember my dad doing this first thing every a.m. (smart man, he was, for listening to Mom). I agree with Mom, and my advice is to get some liquid into your body first thing in the morning: Drink a cup of green tea, a glass of purple grape juice mixed with water, a glass of pomegranate juice mixed with water, or just plain water. Looks like Mom definitely was on to something.

- **Sleep and stroke:** Do you or your significant other snore? If so, you could be at risk for a stroke. According to the American Association of Sleep Medicine (AASM), about 45 percent of Americans snore occasionally and 25 percent snore frequently. Snoring is often a cause of sleep deprivation, not only for the snorer, but for the significant other whose sleep is disturbed. In fact, the

AASM recently reported on a new trend that has emerged in the building industry aimed at providing the spouse with some relief from the loud snoring of his or her partner. Now, instead of being sent to sleep on the living room couch, many partners are sent off to the "snoring room," a second bedroom adjacent to the master bedroom, about twelve feet by twelve feet in size, and equipped with a double bed and chair. However, snoring is more than just annoying in many cases: It is strongly associated with sleep-disordered breathing and sleep apnea. In fact, several studies have shown that obstructive sleep apnea syndrome significantly increases the risk of stroke or death from any cause, and the increase is independent of other risk factors including hypertension.

- **Sleep, obesity, and diabetes:** One unsung reason for the current epidemic of obesity and diabetes in this country may just be the amount of sleep we're getting—or not getting—each night. There is a well-documented relationship between sleep deprivation and high Body Mass Index (BMI). In fact, one study found that the increased BMI was proportional to the decrease in sleep time.

As we sleep our bodies increase the production of leptin, a hormone that suppresses appetite. At the same time we're decreasing the appetite-stimulating hormone grehlin. If your average sleep time is only five hours a night, you produce about 18 percent less leptin and 15 percent more grehlin. So during the hours you're awake you're more likely to be hungrier than normal, especially for foods with high carbohydrate content. You might not think that your sleep habits could affect your food cravings, but, in fact, one study showed that following several days of sleep restriction participants had a 30 percent greater desire for calorie-dense foods like cake and potatoes. The increased high-carb intake added about 350 to 500 calories a day, thus causing weight gain and the potential for obesity. Fatty tissue is also jammed with macrophages, immune system cells that secrete substances that can cause inflammation. Fat is "fire"—it's red hot and smoking! It's not just sitting around doing nothing—it's busy producing inflammatory chemicals, which in turn can react with inflammatory markers made by the liver (such as C-reactive protein). So obesity is characterized by a state of chronic low-grade inflammation.

- **Sleep, cancer, and working the night shift:** In December 2007, the World Health Organization declared shift work as a "possible carcinogen," which puts it in the same category as toxic chemicals such as PCBs. In recent years scientists have been trying to answer the question of why women who work at night seem to be more prone to breast cancer than others. Some research has also shown that men who work at night have a higher rate of prostate cancer.

  The answer may be that working at night disrupts the natural circadian rhythm as well as the secretion of the hormone melatonin, which is normally produced at night. This in turn could increase the release of estrogen by the ovaries. Melatonin is a natural tumor suppressant. Light at night—including artificial light—decreases melatonin production. One theory is that exposure to too much light at night can raise the risk of breast cancer by interfering with the brain's production of tumor-suppressing hormones. People who work under artificial light at night (especially in the blue-light spectrum, which includes computer screens and fluorescent bulbs) have been shown to have lower melatonin levels, which may be the reason their risk of developing cancer is higher.

  Another reason for the higher cancer risk probably is lack of sleep, which makes your immune system vulnerable to attack and less able to fight off tumor growth.

◆ BPH (BENIGN PROSTATE HYPERTROPHY): ANOTHER THING THAT KEEPS MEN UP LATE AT NIGHT ◆

BPH leads to prostate enlargement and urinary tract symptoms (such as decreased flow, the sensation that you can't fully empty your bladder, multiple trips to the bathroom during the night). It's the most common prostate disease in older men—in fact, the majority of men over age fifty are presumed to have some urinary symptoms attributable to BPH.

So what can you do to decrease your risk for this bothersome, sleep-depriving malady?

- Walk two to three hours a week: It can lower your risk by as much as 25 percent
- Chill out: Hostility increases your chance of experiencing the symptoms of BPH
- Watch your waistline: Abdominal obesity raises your risk for BPH (see page 81)
- Keep your fasting blood sugar <100 (see page 110)
- Skip butter and stick margarines, which increase your risk for BPH
- Skip full-fat dairy
- Don't skip fruit: Eating fruit decreases your risk for BPH (see SuperFoods list page 244)
- Lower your red meat consumption and lower your risk (no more than 4 ounces a week)
- If you smoke, stop
- Increase dietary zinc from foods such as pumpkin seeds, green peas, nonfat yogurt, spinach, and skinless turkey breast

We have been overlooking the importance of something we spend about one-third of our lives doing. It seems that many of our current health problems can be at least partially solved in our very own bedrooms—it's so obvious, but it gets little mention in today's 24/7 environment. There is much to learn about the complex subject of sleep, but we don't have to wait any longer to institute the simple solutions listed above. There is no downside to these recommendations. You don't have to worry that sometime in the future headlines will be blaring that getting a good night's sleep is bad for your health. So remember: As I said earlier, the bed is for sleep and sex—but it's also for achieving and maintaining SuperHealth.

STRESS AND INFLAMMATION

There is one more benefit to a good night's sleep that's not yet been mentioned: Sleep is a great stress reliever. Reducing the stress in your life, along with a good night's sleep, can help prevent headaches, back pain, high blood pressure, upset stomach, heart disease, anxiety, and depression, and it can help improve your general health, your energy levels, your skin, your weight, your levels of performance, and your immune system.

We all dream of a stress-free life, a life where it's always summertime and the living is easy, where no one bothers us or pushes us around, where we always make smart decisions, win at card games, and never gain a pound no matter what we eat. A life where everyone we know is healthy and happy and creatively fulfilled. Back in the real world, stress is part of the human condition. Try as you might, you really can't avoid it.

But there are ways you can relieve some of the stress in your life:

- **Deep breathing:** There is nothing like a deep cleansing breath to relieve the stress of everyday living. The best part about it is that it can be done anywhere—at home, at work, in the car, on the playground, in bed—at any time. Deep breathing involves not only the lungs but also the abdomen, or diaphragm. Most of us don't breathe from the diaphragm. Instead, we take shallow breaths from our upper chests, and when stress comes into the picture our breath becomes even shallower. That's not good, as shallow breathing limits the amount of oxygen we take in—which makes us feel even more tense, short of breath, and anxious. When you breathe from your chest, you inhale about a teacup of oxygen. When you breathe from your abdomen, you inhale about a quart of oxygen. The deeper the breath, the greater the calming effect. Breathing from the diaphragm helps you relax quickly, breathe positive energy in, and breathe stress out.

- **Walking meditation:** When most people think of meditation, they imagine being seated in an uncomfortable lotus position with legs crossed like a pretzel. But meditation can be done almost anywhere, in almost any position. You don't have to be seated or still to meditate. In walking meditation you focus on the physicality of each step—the sensation of your feet touching the ground, the rhythm of your breath while moving, and feeling the wind against your face, the sensations of the sun, and the rain; and the sounds of nature and the people around you. One of the best things about walking meditation is that it can be done for very short periods of time and can fit into the few quiet spaces in our lives. Walking from the car into the office in the morning can be an opportunity for a minute's walking meditation, as can walking from your house to your car or to the train or bus, or even walking on a busy city street. The goal is to produce a deep state of relaxation and tranquility while simultaneously enhancing mental focus. And while meditation is often used as a spiritual practice, it is also a powerful stress reliever.

- **Tai chi:** Tai chi, an excellent choice for both balance and flexibility as well as stress relief, is an ancient Chinese martial arts form of meditation with a constant flow of energy and movement that combines mental concentration, slow breathing, and dancelike movements. It consists of gentle physical exercises and stretching in a series of postures or movements that flow one into the next without pausing. Is tai chi better than other exercise at reducing stress? It seems that tai chi is equivalent to brisk walking as far as stress reduction, and multiple studies have reported tai chi to be more highly rewarding, positive, and motivating than many other activities. Tai chi can bring a significant reduction in resting blood pressure, perceived stress, and stress level. Although tai chi was first developed as a martial art, today it is primarily practiced as a way of calming the mind, conditioning the body, and reducing stress. Tai chi is a safe, low-impact option for people of all ages and levels of fitness, including older adults and those recovering from injuries. Once you've learned the moves, you can practice it anywhere, at any time, by yourself, or with others. There are tai chi classes and groups almost everywhere these days, and if you can't find a class near you, there is a wide variety of instructional DVDs you can buy to help you learn on your own.

- **Yoga:** Many of the popular techniques found to reduce stress derive from yoga:
  - controlled breathing
  - meditation
  - physical movement
  - mental imagery
  - stretching

  Yoga brings together the mind, body, and spirit. But whether you use yoga for spiritual transformation or for stress management and physical well-being, the benefits are numerous. While yoga is helpful to people of all ages, it is especially beneficial as you get older because it stretches the body, tones the muscles, and relaxes the mind. Yoga, which literally means "union," originated in India and dates back more than five thousand years. Through the practice of yoga, an individual can gain knowledge about physical, emotional, mental, and spiritual well-being.

  There are many different types of yoga. The most popular type, the one that's taught in most gyms and studios, is hatha yoga, which is usually fairly slow-paced and gentle and can provide a good introduction to the basic yoga poses. The best thing about yoga is that it's good for everyone, no matter what your shape or age. Yoga is so adaptable that even people in a wheelchair can practice it because there are many poses you can do with the upper body.

Just as with tai chi, there are classes and groups almost everywhere these days and a wide variety of instructional DVDs.

You Sexy Thing

Sex is good for you. You probably know that already, but a 2006 study out of Scotland actually proved that sex lowers blood pressure and reduces stress. Researchers studied twenty-four women and twenty-two men who kept records of their sexual activity. Then the researchers subjected them to stressful situations, including public speaking and solving verbal arithmetic problems. Those who had had intercourse had better responses to stress than those who had abstained. Seems like a good way to practice stress reduction, don't you think?

My Personal Stress Reducer

For me the power of prayer is the greatest stress reliever. My mantra is "Trust in God." It has never failed to comfort and calm me. My former agent, the late Al Lowman, taught me that when you get ready to go on TV or radio or give a speech, the last thing you do before you start to speak is say, "God, give me the words." Doing this calms me down, and it works every time. What helps me get through the big stuff and the small is attending religious services, reading the Bible, and exercise. Get me outside with the birds and the bees, and I instantly feel better.

What Is Stress?

Technically speaking, stress is a disruption of homeostasis, which is the ability to maintain a stable condition. Stress is anything that disturbs or interferes with the normal physiological equilibrium of an organism. Stress is tension; it's a state of mental or emotional strain or suspense. You know that expression, "The suspense is killing me ... "? Turns out it's not so far from the truth. It's easy for the stress of modern life to become so intense and continuous that the body will exhaust itself due to its inability to recover or adapt to the stress.

Whatever it is that stresses you out causes a very particular physiological reaction, one that was developed as part of our evolutionary survival skills. It's the fight-or-flight response, an ancient genetic pathway that taught us to fear and run from saber-toothed tigers and cave bears. While the cave bear of the past may have been replaced by your bear of a boss today, the stress response is a normal, healthy, and necessary alarm system—if this were not true, the stress response would not be present in all species, in all cultures, and in all individuals.

When a stressful situation is perceived, the sympathetic nervous system, the part that controls involuntary processes such as heartbeat and breathing, sets off an alarm: Your heart rate increases and your lungs take in more oxygen in order to fuel your muscles should either fight or flight be necessary. Your body goes into full readiness mode.

Next, you go into the resistance phase of stress. The adrenal glands start to draw energy and nutrients from reserves throughout the body. Your metabolism increases, you're in full survival mode, and your senses are heightened as you begin to weigh the level of danger you face and consider your options.

Once the danger has receded, you go into a recovery phase where the body's systems slowly return to normal. The parasympathetic nervous system (the part that when stimulated slows heart rate, lowers blood pressure, and slows breathing) takes over once the "danger" has receded and tells us to "calm down and chill out."

But what happens if you get stuck in one of the first two phases, say when you face the kind of modern stress that follows us all day and well into the night? The body will exhaust itself. It will use up any reserves it might have, and your health will most likely suffer with diseases ranging from ulcers to arthritis, asthma, eczema, depression, and cardiovascular disease. There seem to be two likely pathways for stress to cause and contribute to disease. One is behavioral—people under stress are less likely to exercise, less likely to eat well, less likely to comply with medical treatment, and more likely to suffer from sleep disorders and poor sleep hygiene. The second pathway is physiological: Stress triggers the body's endocrine system, which releases hormones that influence other biological systems, including the immune system, which leaves you more vulnerable to disease.

If you are in a persistent stressful situation, such as a high-pressure job or an unhappy relationship, your body is constantly revved up and ready for a battle. You can't wind down from the tension, and your body never fully returns to a normal relaxed state. Chronic stress appears to blunt the immune response and increase the risk for illness and infection. Studies have shown that people under chronic stress have lower than normal white blood cell counts, are more susceptible to colds and other viruses, take longer to recover from them, and experience worse symptoms than people who do not have high stress levels.

SuperFoods and Stress Relief

People handle stress in many different ways. Some people go home and take a long hot bath. Some go to the gym for a strenuous workout or play a game of softball on the weekends. Others make unhealthy coping choices, such as drugs or alcohol. Often we think we can handle it ourselves and adapt to changing circumstance, and in most ways we do. But for many of us, the first thing we do when we encounter stress is eat.

Stress often triggers the eating of comfort foods—foods high in fat and/or carbohydrates. One of the consequences of this stress-induced eating is that it causes disturbances in a hormone called cholecystokinin (CCK), which is released from the lining of the stomach during the early stages of digestion and which acts as a hunger suppressant. In other words, stress blocks the feeling of satiety, the feeling of being full. When we eat because of stress we eat too many carbs too quickly. We don't give the CCK time to do its job. We gobble down our meals in ten or fifteen minutes, which makes everything we eat fast food. By the time the CCK has a chance to kick in, we're long past satiated and well into "stuffed."

Stress, Serotonin, and Carbohydrate-Rich Foods

Serotonin is a neurotransmitter that helps send messages across synapses in the brain and plays a central role in mood and depression. A decline in activity in serotonin-producing neurons has been associated with disturbances of mood and depression. So a rise in the serotonergic activity in the central nervous system is a good thing because it helps us cope with stress and helps prevent stress-induced depression.

When serotonin levels are at their optimum, we can operate on an even keel without wildly fluctuating mood swings. However, when chronic stress stimulates an overproduction of serotonin, it can lead to a shortage of the supply of this neurotransmitter. As a result, coping, mood, and accuracy of performance deteriorate. Some popular antidepressant drugs such as Prozac work to increase the level of available serotonin in the brain. But you don't need drugs to regulate your serotonin. You do it every day whenever you consume carbohydrates, because they also raise serotonin levels.

The Comfort of Tryptophan

You don't have to understand how serotonin works to know that carbohydrates make you feel better. When you're under stress and your body calls out for comfort food, you don't crave a carrot or a broccoli floret. You want carbs and you want them now. Here's my advice: Instead choose skinless turkey or chicken breast, wild salmon, tuna, soybeans, or sardines, which are rich in tryptophan, the precursor to serotonin.

As you can see, the combination of lack of proper nutrition, lack of exercise, lack of sleep, and too much stress is of great importance to public health. The United States (and the rest of world) is on fire, and not from global warming. Inflammation is on the rise. Picture yourself with smoke and flames constantly burning inside you until you get too hot to touch. It's almost as if you've gotten internal heatstroke. The treatment for heatstroke is to immerse the patient in ice. To put out the heat of inflammation, you need to wrap yourself in the ice treatment of the SuperHealth diet and lifestyle. For the complete Week 4 Planner, see page 304.

◆ MEET JOHN CARVER ◆

Attitude Is Everything

"Getting old is not for sissies," says John Carver, now well into his seventies. "You've got to have the right attitude about everything. My philosophy is: Control the controllables. If you can't control it, don't worry about it."

Carver is a native Californian who, when asked if he ate well as a child, laughs and says, "Absolutely not. I grew up eating what I could get. My mom would cook for us, but if there was a box of cookies around, it wouldn't last very long. And when I grew up, I didn't do much better. Every day for lunch I used to have a Burger King combo because it was the closest place to the office. But not anymore."

He doesn't eat that way anymore because he's had two heart attacks, and he currently has four stents (tiny metal devices used to keep collapsed arteries open). Now he eats healthy foods, with the caveat that if he has a craving for something like Kentucky Fried, he'll have one drumstick and that's enough. And his condition hasn't stopped him from getting out and about. He works out at the gym three days a week, and he also volunteers at the local cardiac treatment center. He sees people come in for their postoperative treatment and "they're scared to death," he says. "But I give them a friendly greeting and show them the ropes. They quietly say to me, 'I just had a heart attack,' and I say, 'Oh yeah? I've had two. And look at me!' "

The secret to life is to help other people, says Carver. "When you help people, you get more out of it than they do. When I was a child, a minister told me, 'A person never stands so tall as when he stoops to help a child.' That's stayed with me all these years. It doesn't literally mean a child; it means someone who is in need. I've based my life on that. I'll never tell you to change your whole lifestyle, but I will say watch your diet, get plenty of exercise, and be aware that this could be your last day on earth. Make sure that you have peace with God and that you're happy. You'll live a lot longer that way."

7

Step 5: Keep Up Appearances

For your basics, see the SuperHealth Food Pyramid, page 19 (for your bonus see below)

Week 5 SuperFoods:

Dark chocolate	Tomatoes
Avocados	Pumpkin
Oranges	Tea
Dried fruit	

Don't you want to look as great as you can for as long as you can? Don't you want to prevent wrinkles and age spots, get rid of rough, dry skin, and reduce the risk of skin cancer? Wouldn't you like your skin to have a nice even tone, to give you a smoother, more radiant, younger appearance? All of that is possible without a lot of effort on your part. Just include in your diet some of the foods in this week's SuperFoods list (how hard is it to have a bite of dark chocolate now and again?), keep that exercise routine going, add in a few SuperNutrients, and in no time you'll not only be looking great, you'll be feeling healthier as well.

The visible signs of aging often appear well before we're ready for them. However, it turns out that we can get a lot of clues about our insides by studying our outsides. What can you tell from bleeding gums? What can you glean from poor posture? What does dull, wrinkled skin tell you? You don't have to be a psychic to get hints for the future just from studying a person's appearance.

It's easy to understand that your health affects your appearance, but is the opposite true? In most cases it is. If your teeth and gums are in bad shape, it's a pretty good bet that your cardiovascular system and lungs are in bad shape, too. If you have problems sitting or standing up straight, your bones and muscles will let you down when you need them most (to prevent a fall). And if your skin shows signs of premature aging (wrinkles, sags, bags, discoloration, rough spots) and sun damage, your insides probably reflect the same. So though some may claim that putting extra effort into the care and maintenance of the only body you have is self-indulgent, I say it's really about self-preservation.

For instance, is your skin dull and sallow? Or does it have a rosy glow? If you want to look your best and add more color to your outside, add more color to your inside. All the color you find in the skin of fruits and vegetables you eat ends up in your skin, too. There's a definite correlation between how skin ages and the food you eat. The more polyphenols (found in berries, nuts and seeds, tea, and fruits and veggies in general) you consume, the fewer wrinkles you get. The nutrients that give a blueberry its smooth skin will give you smooth skin as well—at the same time giving you all the other health benefits the mighty blueberry bestows.

Outward signs like dark circles under the eyes and red, puffy gums mean that your body is in an inflammatory state, which can fuel the onset of cardiovascular disease. You are generating too many free radicals in your system and are short on antioxidants. Your circulatory system is most likely not up to par, and every part of your body demands good circulation to give you SuperHealth. Those outward signs are a good thing because they let us know that things are going awry inside, and we can make the healthy changes and choices—

both dietary and lifestyle—that will help us live many more years.

And the truth is, the ultimate compliment in life is when you tell people your age and they say, "But you look so much younger!" There is nothing more attractive than the glow of good health. Everyone wants to look good no matter what their age. The happier you are when you look in the mirror, the better you feel. And the better you feel, the more confident you are. The more confident you are, the more you look forward to a happy, healthy future, and the more likely you are to take better care of yourself and the way you look.

Paying attention to the way we look both optimizes appearance and provides benefits that are far more than skin deep. Of course, taking care of your skin starts with proper nutrition, exercise (which promotes good blood flow), sleep (a natural anti-inflammatory), and stress reduction (another anti-inflammatory). All of those factors will naturally help us look healthier and more vibrant, which automatically translates into looking younger. When we're young, we have a healthy supply of growth factors, enzymes, and hormones to keep us looking firm and fit, but this supply diminishes as we age. Combine this fact with less sleep, more stress, and harmful lifestyle choices such as eating, drinking, smoking, and tanning too much, and we've got the perfect formula for accelerated aging.

The way to slow down that aging process is to follow the SuperHealth program of nutrition and lifestyle choices so that you are able to replenish and revitalize those hormones and enzymes necessary to keep you both looking and feeling good for as long as possible.

It starts with the skin because that's what people see first when they look at you. You can hide a lot of flaws from other people underneath your clothes, but unless you're covered from head to foot, you can't hide your skin. All the expensive skin-care products in the world won't achieve or maintain healthy skin without help from your diet. You've got to take care of your skin from the inside out if you want to look and feel great.

The SuperFoods featured in this chapter are included here primarily because they help increase the sun protective factor (SPF) of the skin from the inside out. The nutrients in these foods travel from the vascular system into the skin and protect it against damage from the sun.

Dark Chocolate

Recommended amount: About 100 calories of dark chocolate daily, adjusting your calorie intake and exercise appropriately

What if there was an edible sunscreen that was both delicious and effective? What if it looked, smelled, and tasted like chocolate? What if it was chocolate? Well, it is! Chocolate is good for the skin. Actually, it's the polyphenols in chocolate that are good for the skin. But it's not just any chocolate; it's dark chocolate that contains skin-health-promoting nutrients. Researchers now believe that flavonoids (a type of polyphenols found in cocoa beans, red wine, tea, cranberries, and other fruits) absorb UV light and help protect and increase blood flow to the skin, improving its appearance. In one German study a group of women were given either a high-flavonol chocolate drink or a low-flavonol chocolate drink for twelve weeks. They were told to continue their normal dietary habits, but sunbathing and tanning beds were forbidden. Three times during the study participants were exposed to enough UV radiation to redden the skin. Researchers found that the group that had received the high-flavonol dark-chocolate beverage had a 25 percent reduction in skin response to the ultraviolet radiation by week twelve, while the low-flavonol group showed no difference in response. In the high-flavonol group the women's skin was moister, smoother, less scaly, and not as red after exposure to ultraviolet light.

The amount of flavonols in chocolate can vary widely depending on how the cocoa beans are harvested and processed. The higher the amount of cocoa solids, the more polyphenols the chocolate will contain. Look for at least 70 percent cocoa solids—you will find the percentage of cocoa solids on the labels of most good chocolate bars.

Avocados

Recommended amount: ⅓ to ½ of an avocado multiple times weekly

Sidekicks: asparagus, artichokes, extra virgin olive oil

One of the most nutrient-dense and calorie-dense foods available, avocados are high in fiber and, ounce for ounce, top the charts among all fruits for folate (folic acid, one of the B vitamins), potassium, vitamin E, and magnesium. Magnesium is an essential nutrient for healthy bones as well as the cardiovascular system; it also helps in the prevention of type 2 diabetes and seems to delay the aging of our cells. Avocados provide more magnesium than the twenty most commonly eaten fruits.

Research has found that certain nutrients are absorbed better when eaten with avocados. In one study participants who ate a salad containing avocados absorbed 20 percent more carotenoids (a group of nutrients that includes lycopene and beta-carotene) from the tomatoes or carrots in the salad than those who ate a salad that didn't include avocados.

Avocados are the best fruit source of vitamin E, an essential vitamin that protects against many diseases and helps maintains overall health, but it is important for skin health, as it helps to neutralize the free radicals produced by UV radiation. For a terrific guacamole recipe, see page 281. One of my favorite ways to eat avocados is to spread half of an avocado over a slice of whole grain toast, and top it off with La Victoria Mild Red Taco Sauce. This is about a 240-calorie snack, so keep that in mind if you're watching your weight. To prevent the unused half of the avocado from turning brown, squeeze some lemon juice over it and place it in a zip-top plastic bag. Guess who taught me that tip— you're right, it was Mom again.

Oranges

Recommended amount: 1 medium orange, ½ cup orange juice daily

Sidekicks: lemons, white and pink grapefruit, kumquats, tangerines, limes

It's ironic that the orange, a fruit with such wrinkly skin, can help prevent us from getting our own wrinkles. Vitamin C is essential for making collagen, a natural protein found in the connective tissues that support the skin and help keep the skin elastic. In one of the first studies to examine the impact of nutrients from foods rather than supplements on skin aging, researchers reported that people who ate plenty of vitamin C–rich foods had fewer wrinkles than people whose diets contained little of the vitamin.

Human beings cannot manufacture vitamin C in our bodies and we therefore need constant replenishment of this vitamin from dietary sources. A single navel orange, only 64 calories, provides almost one-quarter of my daily dietary vitamin C recommendation of 350 milligrams or more (more on this later in the chapter). Many of the phytonutrients and fiber are in the orange pulp, so if you're buying orange juice, get the kind with the pulp. While oranges are an extremely rich source of vitamin C, they also provide more than 170 different phytochemicals and more than 60 flavonoids. These nutrients working together have anti-inflammatory, antitumor, antiviral, antiallergenic, and blood-clot-inhibiting properties. And don't forget to eat a bit of the peel (or include some zest in your favorite recipes) to decrease LDL "bad" cholesterol, glucose, and insulin levels, and to help prevent skin cancer.

Dried Fruit

Recommended amounts: 2 heaping tablespoons, three to four times a week

Sidekicks: raisins, dates, prunes, and dried figs, apricots, blueberries, cranberries, cherries, currants

When the weather gets cold and you're looking for fresh fruit at your local market, the pickin's might just be slimmer than you'd like. That's the time to go for some dried fruit, which can be a tasty source of health-promoting nutrients, as the nutrients in dried fruits are more concentrated if you measure them by volume. In fact, dried fruits also have a greater fiber content, increased shelf life, and significantly greater polyphenol content than fresh fruit (except for vitamin C; there's very little of it in dried fruit). This is a great way to boost your skin health by getting in those polyphenols all year round. One of the advantages of dried fruits is that they're portable, so they're easy to include in a brown-bag lunch or as a snack at work.

While dried fruit selection used to be limited to raisins, dates, and prunes, you can now find dried blueberries, cranberries, cherries, currants, apricots, and figs in most supermarkets and health food stores. Check the package labels and avoid dried fruit that has been sweetened with high-fructose corn syrup. I prefer to buy organic dried fruit because any pesticides that may have been sprayed onto the fresh fruit get concentrated when the fruit is dried.

The most nutrient-dense dried fruits are apricots and figs, followed by plums, raisins, dates, and cranberries. You can add dried fruit to oatmeal in the last five minutes of cooking and to quick breads, cookies, and other baked goods. And, of course, a small box of raisins makes a great lunchbox snack.

Tomatoes

Recommended amounts: 1 serving of processed tomatoes, such as 1 to 2 tablespoons of tomato paste (see page 271 for more suggestions), or sidekicks listed below, a day, and multiple servings a week of fresh tomatoes

Sidekicks: watermelon, pink grapefruit, red-fleshed papayas, Japanese persimmons, strawberry guavas

One of the reasons tomatoes are considered a Super-

Food is because they contain lycopene, another important carotenoid. About 85 percent of lycopene in the Western diet is obtained from tomatoes, and the best place to find it is in tomato paste. Tomato paste in particular has a very high concentration of bioavailable lycopene because cooking releases lycopene from plant cell walls. Lycopene from fruit sources, such as the tomato sidekicks above, is readily bioavailable without cooking or processing.

A study conducted by the BBC Science and Nature in London was done to establish whether eating tomato paste could help protect the skin from UV damage and UV-induced reddening. Twenty-three women who sunburned easily took part in the experiment. Half of them were asked to eat 55 grams of tomato paste every day for twelve weeks (giving them 16 milligrams of lycopene— you can get that much lycopene from a cup of tomato sauce, a cup of tomato soup or tomato juice, or 6 tablespoons of ketchup). Participants were then exposed to a range of UV radiation, and researchers compared the damage done to those who ate tomatoes and those who didn't. After twelve weeks of eating tomato paste daily, the women were tested again. Those who had consumed the tomato paste showed a 30 percent increase in skin protection. That doesn't mean that you should stop using sunblock and start eating tomatoes, but it does mean that adding cooked tomato products to your diet can be an important boost to your SuperHealth and SuperSkin program. If you're going for fresh tomatoes, you might want to choose cherry tomatoes—they have the highest antioxidant amounts per mouthful because of their thick skin.

There are a small number of people who have an inflammatory response to nightshade vegetables such as tomatoes and eggplant. If you are in that number, stick to the lycopene-rich sidekicks: watermelon, pink grapefruit, Japanese persimmons, red-fleshed papayas, and strawberry guavas.

Pumpkin

Recommended amounts: ½ cup, five to seven days a week

Sidekicks: carrots, butternut squash, sweet potatoes, orange bell peppers

Of all of the phytonutrients, the most information is known about the carotenoids. The carotenoid family includes alpha-carotene, beta-carotene, b-cryptoxanthin, lutein, lycopene, and zeaxanthin. Two of the carotenoids that are in rich supply in pumpkins—beta-carotene and alpha-carotene—are particularly powerful.

Pumpkin (either fresh or canned), carrots (raw, cooked, or juiced), and butternut squash are all excellent sources of both alpha-carotene and beta-carotene, both of which provide protection against UV light and help to reduce photosensitivity, which promotes skin renewal and protects the skin from sun damage. To optimize the carotenoid "glow" in your skin, these three SuperFoods are a must. Pumpkins and its sidekicks are rich in antioxidants, including phytochemicals, vitamins, and minerals, which protect, nourish, and moisturize the skin.

Absolute musts: If there's only one pumpkin sidekick you add for the week, or if you're traveling and can't control your diet, my recommendation is one 8-ounce glass of organic carrot juice most days. You might be surprised to know how easy it is to find—most juicing places can make it for you and most grocery stores will have it in their health food section. Some of my favorite brands of carrot juice are Evolution Organic Carrot Juice, Odwalla Carrot Juice, Naked Carrot Juice, and Bolthouse Farms Organic Carrot Juice (www.bolthouse.com).

> ### Slim Down for Healthy Skin
>
> One way to improve your skin (as well as your health) is to lose weight. That's because if you're heavy, the carotenoids that would pass into your skin cells and protect you from sun damage get sucked into fat cells instead and just sit there where they can do you no good. So shed some pounds and gain some carotenoids!

Tea

Recommended amounts: 4 or more cups daily

Tea is rich in antioxidant flavonoids, especially one called epigallocatechin-3-gallate, better known as EGCG. EGCG is a catechin, a subclass of flavonoids. Scientists have calculated that the tea plant ranks as one of the highest in total flavonoid content. FYI: Decaffeinated tea loses about 15 to 20 percent of its antioxidants, and at least with skin cancer and prostate cancer, caffeinated tea seems to be more efficacious than decaffeinated tea in preventing those cancers.

Since the 1990s hundreds of studies have been performed suggesting that tea possesses anticancer effects. Most of the research on tea has focused on green tea, but it is known that black tea also offers beneficial effects to skin and other body organs.

It seems the most important SuperNutrient in tea is polyphenols. Tea polyphenols possess antioxidant, anti-inflammatory, and anticarcinogenic properties. Several recent studies have shown that the polyphenols in tea are effective cancer fighters. In one study, University of Alabama researchers found that the EGCG in green tea prevents UV radiation–induced suppression of the immune system, which has been considered a risk factor for the development of skin cancer. In 2006 British researchers found that tea extracts can help damaged skin that has been affected by UV radiation by working at the cellular level of the skin and reducing inflammation by inhibiting inflammatory pathways. Another study showed that having a cup of tea—green or black, hot or cold—every day can help lower the risk of two common forms of skin cancer: basal-cell and squamous-cell carcinoma.

Tea is also known to contain fluoride, an important mineral for bone development. When researchers at the University of Cambridge in England examined the tea-drinking habits and bone densities of more than 1,200 elderly British women, they found that tea drinkers had significantly stronger bones than non-tea drinkers. Tea is also often used in topical skin-care treatments, and it is currently being studied as an effective treatment for more severe skin complaints from the destructive effects of sunlight. I personally use tea as a topical skin treatment almost every day. After I use a tea bag, I squeeze it dry and wipe it over my face like a sponge, especially over my nose, forehead, and cheeks (more than 50 percent of all skin cancers on the body are on the middle of the face). I just love the feeling of those flavonoids going to work to keep me healthy and looking good!

Is the Tea You're Drinking Really Tea?

True teas, including white, green, black, and oolong tea, are all derived from the leaves or buds of the tea tree, *Camellia sinensis*. Green tea is not healthier than black tea or oolong tea. All varieties of tea contain similar amounts of antioxidants, although they are of different types. They all provide health benefits. The different tea varieties are formulated by allowing the leaves to oxidize to different degrees and at times combining them with spices, herbs, or fruit extracts. It is important to note that the term "herbal tea" traditionally refers to infusions of fruits or herbs and typically contains no actual tea.

Red tea (rooibos), which is grown in South Africa, is

caffeine-free and contains a wide array of phytonutrients. To date it is one of the only herbal teas with a significant body of scientific literature to support the health claims associated with its consumption. (Rooibos has been shown to be antimutagenic, anticarcinogenic, anti-inflammatory, and antiviral. And, like true tea, it helps to give you strong bones and teeth because of its calcium, manganese, and fluoride content.)

Week 5: Keep Up Appearances Daily Food Planner

The chart below is an example of how you can add this week's foods to your SuperHealth program. It doesn't mean these are the only foods you should eat for the week, they are just suggestions for what should be added to your diet. Feel free to mix and match foods and days to your heart's content. And don't forget to have at least one cup of tea every day.

	Food Suggestion	Daily Servings
Day 1	Dark chocolate	100 calories
	Avocado	⅓ avocado
	Orange	1 medium (1 baseball)
	Raisins	2 heaping tablespoons (heaping shot glass)
	Tomato	1 medium (1 baseball)
	Pumpkin	½ cup (½ baseball)
	Tea	4 cups
Day 2	Asparagus	½ cup (½ baseball)
	Pink grapefruit	1 medium (1 baseball)
	Tomato paste	2 tablespoons (1 shot glass)
	Carrots	½ cup (½ baseball)
	Tea	4 cups
Day 3	Dark chocolate	100 calories
	EVOO	2 tablespoons (1 shot glass)

(continued)

	Food Suggestion	**Daily Servings**
Day 3 (*cont.*)	Blueberries	1 cup (1 baseball)
	Tomato	1 medium (1 baseball)
	Orange bell pepper	½ cup (½ baseball)
	Tea	4 cups
Day 4	Dark chocolate	100 calories
	Artichoke	½ cup (½ baseball)
	Kumquats	2 small kumquats
	Tomato paste	2 tablespoons (1 shot glass)
	Butternut squash	½ cup (½ baseball)
	Tea	4 cups
Day 5	Avocado	⅓ avocado
	Orange juice	½ cup (4 ounces)
	Dried cranberries	2 heaping tablespoons (heaping shot glass)
	Watermelon	1 cup (1 baseball)
	Sweet potato	½ cup (½ baseball)
	Tea	4 cups
Day 6	Dark chocolate	100 calories
	Lemon juice	½ cup (4 ounces)
	Currants	2 heaping tablespoons (heaping shot glass)
	Tomato paste	2 tablespoons (1 shot glass)
	Pumpkin	½ cup (½ baseball)
	Tea	4 cups
Day 7	Dark chocolate	100 calories
	EVOO	2 tablespoons (1 shot glass)
	Orange	1 medium (1 baseball)
	Persimmon	1 medium (1 baseball)
	Carrots	½ cup (½ baseball)
	Tea	4 cups

EXERCISE AND APPEARANCE

Controlling your diet isn't the only way to keep up your appearance. Exercise, too, plays an important role in how you look and feel. It increases circulation, which delivers nutrients and allows for a restful sleep, giving the skin a chance to rejuvenate. And of course, it increases bone and muscle strength. Researchers are now finding that exercise can have dramatic effects on acne-prone skin, because it mediates the production of testosterone-related hormones such as DHEA and DHT that are part of acne flare-ups. One of the reasons for this is that the production of these hormones from the adrenal glands is related to stress. The more stress you're under, the more of these hormones you produce, which is why we always seem to get breakouts just before an important event. Exercise reduces stress, which tends to quiet the adrenal glands.

Exercise has also been shown to protect against the growth of skin tumors. A group of researchers exposed mice to UVB radiation for sixteen weeks. Half the mice had running wheels in their cages, while the other half did not. The mice who exercised had far fewer tumors, and the tumors they did develop were smaller and took longer to form.

So add skin health to the long list of the benefits of exercise, and continue the exercise portion of the SuperHealth program:

- **Walk the Walk:** Increase your walking time to at least 25 minutes, five to six days a week. If you counted your steps last week via your pedometer, increase your amount by 500 steps for this week. So if you started last week with 4,000 steps each day, your goal for this week is 4,500 steps each day.
- **Dr. Steve's Power Stairs Workout:** Increase the number of times you walk up and down the stairs in your home or office. If you were doing 7 minutes last week, try for two to four days of 10 min-

utes each this week and increase the speed at which you walk.

- **Heel to Fanny:** Stand on stairs or an elevated area (this can be done on a flat surface as well), and hold on to the railing or the wall keeping your knees together. The left leg remains straight. With your right leg beginning in a straight position, bring your right heel to your fanny. You may not be able to touch your fanny, but take it as far as you can and hold it there for 4 seconds, then let it down slowly. Increase to 3 sets of 20 with each leg three to four days a week. This builds strength in the hamstrings, those big muscles in the backs of the thighs.

- **Sit-up/Crunch:** Lie on your back with your knees bent and your feet flat on the floor in front of you. Lie on an exercise mat or carpet rather than a hard floor to prevent back strain. Your feet should be as wide apart as your hips. Place your arms crossed on your chest and keep your chin pointing upward. Curl up and forward so that your head, neck, and shoulder blades lift off the floor. Pause for a count of one, then slowly lower your shoulder blades, neck, and head to the starting position. Increase to 3 sets of 30, three days a week.

- **Isometric Curl:** Hold on to the back of the steering wheel (while at a stop sign or signal) at the five o'clock and seven o'clock positions with your palms facing toward you and your arms bent. This can also be done by grabbing the edge of a desk or table, palms facing up, elbows at your sides, shoulders down. The idea is to attempt to bring your hands up toward your shoulders (you won't actually be able to do it—the point is to get the resistance). Hold the position for 10 to 20 seconds and repeat 20 times using both arms. This helps to tone the biceps and the front part of the shoulder muscles. For maximum benefit, vary the amount of arm bend slightly for each rep, as this strengthens the muscle at varying degrees of use. Make sure to keep your shoulders down and back. Do this two to four times a week.

- **Isometric Extension:** Again, this is a nonmovement form of strengthening. This time you're pushing against the steering wheel, desk, or any other immobile surface, with the heel of your hand and your fingers pointing down. Try to extend or straighten your arms, using your body weight to resist. Hold the position for 10 to 20 seconds and repeat 20 times using both arms. This helps to tone the triceps (backs of the arms). Do this two to four times a week.

- **Tennis Ball Squeeze:** Keep a tennis ball or other type of ball, soft or hard, at your desk, in the car, or around the house. Squeeze at least 20 times a day (more if you want). Squeezing the ball and holding it for a count of 20 can actually help lower your blood pressure. It's a good one to do while you're on the phone during a stressful conversation—stress is a major source of inflammation.

- **Stand Up/Sit Down:** This is one you can do anywhere, as many times as you want. Simply get up from your chair (do not use a chair with wheels) without using your arms to push you up. Do not lean forward to get momentum; the object is to use your leg muscles. Then sit slowly all the way back down into the chair, focusing on your quads, the muscles at the fronts of your thighs. As your quad muscles get stronger, go down until you're almost but not quite sitting and then come back up. This is another good exercise to do while you're talking on the phone. Repeat as many times as you like.

- **Wall Sit**: If your legs are weak or the Stand Up/Sit Down exercise is hard on your knees, start off with a Wall Sit instead. Place your butt, back, and shoulders flat against the wall, with your feet about hip-distance apart about 1.5 feet away from the wall. Slide your back down the wall so your knees are bending. Go as low as you can go to start (the goal is to form a 90-degree angle with your bent knees—if you do it right, your body should look like it's sitting in an invisible chair). Hold this for a count of 5, and slide back up the wall. Repeat with your feet straight ahead, and again with your toes facing inward. As you get stronger, slide farther down the wall until your legs are at a 90-degree angle and you are holding for a count of 10. Repeat as many times as you like.

- **Steering Wheel Squeeze:** While parked or at a red light, grip the steering wheel so that your hands are horizontally across from each other (at the three o'clock and nine o'clock positions). Your elbows are out and your arms should be forming a "C" shape. Try to push your hands together against the steering wheel—imagine that you're trying to close the "C" shape of your arms into an "O" shape. Hold this for 5 to 10 seconds, then let go. Repeat 15 times. This is great for building forearms, biceps, and shoulder muscles. You can try it outside the car, too: Grab either side of the back of a chair and try to push your arms from a "C" into an "O." Do this two to four times a week.

- **Bicep Curl:** Stand with your feet about hip-width apart as you hold a light weight in each hand in front of the thighs. Choose a weight that allows you to easily do 3 sets of 10 curls (you can also use cans of soup or vegetables if you don't have weights). Your grip should be underhand (palms facing upward). Squeeze your biceps and bend your arms, curling the weights up toward your shoulders. Keep your elbows stationary and at the sides of your body and bring the weights only as high as you can without moving your elbows. Slowly lower the weights, keeping a slight bend in the elbows at the bottom (don't lock the joints; try to keep tension on the muscle). If you can easily do 3 sets of 10, add 5 pounds of weight. Repeat for 3 sets of 10 reps, two to three times a week.

- **Tricep Extension:** From a standing position with your feet about hip-width apart, hold a light weight (or can) in your right hand. Bend forward so that your upper torso is perpendicular to the floor, keeping your right arm straight at your side. Bend and raise your elbow up toward the ceiling until your arm is at a right angle at your side, then extend your arm backward until it's straight. Hold and lower slowly. If you can easily do 2 sets of 10, add 2.5 to 5 pounds of weight. Repeat for 2 sets of 10, then repeat with your left arm. Do this two to four times a week.

This week, add these few more exercises:

- **Waist Twist:** Standing with your legs about shoulder-width apart, place a broom with a long handle or a dowel that's about six feet long behind your neck. Grasp the broom with both hands, palms facing forward. Start out with your entire body facing forward, then without moving the lower half of your body, twist from your waist as far as you can to your right. Go back to center, then twist as far as you can to your left. Repeat for 3 sets of 20, three to four days a week.
- **Side Bends:** Standing with your legs about shoulder-width apart, place a broom with a long handle or a dowel that's about six feet long behind your neck. Grasp the broom with both hands, palms facing forward. Start out with your entire body facing forward, then without moving the lower half of your body, bend at your waist as far as you can to your right so that one end of the dowel is facing the floor and the other is facing the ceiling. Go back to center, then bend as far as you can to your left. Repeat for 3 sets of 20, three to four days a week.
- **Bicycle:** Lie on your back on an exercise mat or carpet. Lift your legs up in the air, then bend your knees so that your calves are at a right angle to your thighs. Keep your arms on the floor at your sides to stabilize your body, then begin to "pedal" as if you were riding a bike. Bicycle for 30 seconds, three to four times a week.
- **Platysma Rock:** Here's a good way to get rid of

that "turkey neck" we all hate. The muscle that runs from your clavicle to your jaw and the skin around your mouth is the platysma muscle. Flex that muscle by keeping your head at its normal, upright position while using your face and neck muscles to pull your lower lip down away from upper lip, exposing your lower teeth entirely. Try to make the corners of your lips point downward. You should be making an inverted smile or grimacing face that tenses the muscles in your neck. Hold this face for 5 seconds, then release. Repeat 10 times or more a day. This is something you can easily do in the car, at your desk, or while watching your favorite TV show.

Week 5: Keep Up Appearances Daily Exercise Planner

The chart below is an example of how you can add this week's exercises to your SuperHealth program.

	Exercise	Set Reminders
Day 1	Walk	25 minutes
	Power Stairs	10 minutes
	Heel to Fanny	3 sets of 20
	Isometric Curl	20 times with both arms; hold for 20 seconds
	Isometric Extension	20 times with both arms; hold for 20 seconds
	Ball Squeeze	20 times
	Steering Wheel Squeeze	3 sets of 15
	Waist Twist	3 sets of 20
	Side Bends	3 sets of 20
	Platysma Rock	10 times
Day 2	Walk	25 minutes
	Heel to Fanny	3 sets of 20
	Sit-up/Crunch	3 sets of 30
	Isometric Curl	20 times with both arms; hold for 20 seconds
	Isometric Extension	20 times with both arms; hold for 20 seconds

Exercise	**Set Reminders**
Bicep Curl	3 sets of 10; add weight
Tricep Extension	3 sets of 10; add weight
Bicycle	30 seconds

Day 3	Exercise	Set Reminders
	Walk	25 minutes
	Power Stairs	10 minutes
	Ball Squeeze	20 times
	Stand Up/Sit Down/Wall Sit	Unlimited times
	Steering Wheel Squeeze	3 sets of 15
	Waist Twist	3 sets of 20
	Side Bends	3 sets of 20
	Platysma Rock	10 times

Day 4	Exercise	Set Reminders
	Walk	25 minutes
	Heel to Fanny	3 sets of 20
	Sit-up/Crunch	3 sets of 30
	Isometric Curl	20 times with both arms; hold for 20 seconds
	Isometric Extension	20 times with both arms; hold for 20 seconds
	Ball Squeeze	20 times
	Stand Up/Sit Down/Wall Sit	Unlimited times
	Bicycle	30 seconds

Day 5	Exercise	Set Reminders
	Walk	25 minutes
	Power Stairs	10 minutes
	Isometric Curl	20 times with both arms; hold for 20 seconds
	Isometric Extension	20 times with both arms; hold for 20 seconds
	Ball Squeeze	20 times
	Bicep Curl	3 sets of 10; add weight
	Tricep Extension	3 sets of 10; add weight
	Waist Twist	3 sets of 20
	Side Bends	5 sets of 20
	Platysma Rock	10 times

Day 6	Exercise	Set Reminders
	Walk	25 minutes
	Heel to Fanny	3 sets of 20
	Sit-up/Crunch	3 sets of 30
	Ball Squeeze	20 times

(continued)

	Exercise	Set Reminders
Day 6 (*cont.*)	Stand Up/Sit Down/Wall Sit	Unlimited times
	Steering Wheel Squeeze	3 sets of 15
	Bicycle	30 seconds
Day 7	Walk	25 minutes
	Power Stairs	10 minutes
	Isometric Curl	20 times with both arms; hold for 20 seconds
	Isometric Extension	20 times with both arms; hold for 20 seconds
	Bicep Curl	3 sets of 10; add weight
	Tricep Extension	3 sets of 10; add weight
	Waist Twist	3 sets of 20
	Side Bends	3 sets of 20
	Platysma Rock	10 times

YOUR PEARLY WHITES

Although there isn't 100 percent agreement among experts on this topic, most agree that without healthy gums our pearly whites won't be around for the long haul and neither will we. Even as far back as the seventh century B.C., the Assyrians considered the effect of oral health on the rest of the body, which just goes to prove that as for so many things in science, what's new news is really old news: Inflamed gums equals inflammation throughout the body. Healthy gums equals a healthy heart and brain.

According to the American Academy of Periodontology, people with periodontal disease are almost twice as likely to have coronary artery disease as people with healthy gums. Periodontal disease is a chronic bacterial infection characterized by gingivitis (gum inflammation, bleeding, redness, tenderness, and sensitivity) and periodontitis (inflammation of the soft tissue anchoring the teeth into your jawbone). Periodontitis is characterized by inflammation that extends into the soft tissue and bone that supports the teeth. If left untreated, periodontal disease can result in the formation of pockets around the teeth caused by the destruction of the attachment of gums to teeth and teeth to the part of the jaw that holds the teeth. Eventually this can lead to tooth loss.

Neither periodontal disease nor tooth loss is inevitable. A good regimen of dental hygiene can go a long way toward saving your gums and teeth. But so can a healthy diet. A recent study of more than 11,000 adults showed that there is an inverse relationship between the amount of antioxidants in the blood and the risk of periodontal disease. In other words, the more antioxidants—especially where levels of vitamin C are concerned—the lower your risk of having periodontal disease (a whopping 62 percent lower risk for people who have never smoked). And if you can lower your risk of periodontal disease, you also lower your risk not only of heart disease but of stroke and of type 2 diabetes as well.

This information about healthy gums and your overall health may give you a whole new way at looking at yourself and others. Good-looking pearly whites and gums represent a lot more than just a pleasing cosmetic appearance. Healthy gums and healthy teeth are also effective, easy-to-see markers of how your body is aging and how close you are to SuperHealth. Here are some suggestions about how to have and maintain healthy teeth and gums:

- **Swish your tea:** Rinsing your mouth with tea multiple times a day helps to prevent gingivitis. Even if you brush and floss regularly, your mouth is filled with millions of bacteria constantly on the move. While some bacteria are harmless, others can attack the teeth and gums. Harmful bacteria are contained in a colorless sticky film called plaque, the cause of gum disease. If plaque is allowed to build up on the teeth, ultimately it will irritate the gums and cause bleeding. Eventually this plaque buildup will destroy bone and connective tissue, so teeth can often become loose and may have to be removed. One step you can take to fight plaque is to rinse your mouth with tea multiple times a day. It seems that several compounds found in tea are capable of killing or suppressing growth and acid production of cavity-causing bacteria. Tea has also been shown to affect a bacterial enzyme that is responsible for converting sugars into the sticky matrix material that plaque uses to adhere to teeth. Tea also provides prebiotic food to stimulate the growth of healthy bacteria in the mouth—so it kills the "bad guys" and promotes the growth of the "good guys." So the next time you're drinking a cup of tea, don't just swallow it down. Swish it around in your mouth for fifteen to twenty seconds so it gets a chance to help break down the harmful plaque and promote the healthy bacteria that help your teeth stay healthy and intact (of course, this is an adjunct to your regular tooth-health routine, not a substitute for it).

- **Eat your raisins:** Tea is not the only bacteria fighter for your mouth. It seems that a phytochemical in raisins called oleanolic acid inhibits the growth of two species of oral bacteria that cause cavities and periodontal disease. So if you're looking for a sweet snack, a mini-box of raisins (about ¾ ounce) might be the perfect solution.

- **Floss twice a day:** I know, you've heard this before. But it has to be said again, because although brushing and flossing are equally important, brushing eliminates only the plaque from the surfaces of the teeth that the brush can reach. Flossing, on the other hand, removes plaque from in between the teeth and under the gum line. Floss should be like your reading glasses when you're over forty—stash some at your desk, in your car, in your purse or briefcase. Every time you floss your heart sends back a message saying thank you.

- **Use an electric toothbrush:** Most dentists agree

that electric toothbrushes that use an oscillating rotating motion, such as the Braun Oral-B and the Crest SpinBrush Pro, are more effective at reducing plaque than manual brushing. Use it twice a day and brush for two minutes every time.

- **Allow yourself the time you need for good dental hygiene:** Don't rush through your morning and evening routine. Take good care of your teeth and gums and they will take good care of you—they may even save your life.

THE SUPERHEALTH APPROACH TO AGING SKIN

Some people just naturally look great no matter what their age. It's in their genes. Others may not have the genes, but they've taken great care of themselves over the years and it's very hard to tell just how old they are. And still others wear their whole life story on their face—every line and wrinkle tells a tale of tough times and/or a lifetime of bad habits. Whichever category you're in, there's no escaping the fact that as you get older, you face a gradual decline in those factors that give your skin the look and health of youth. However, as you'll find out, there is evidence that eating, and in some cases topically applying specific foods or their components, may play a role in keeping your skin healthier and younger looking. Skin is your largest organ system, so it does deserve some attention.

SuperNutrients for Skin and Health

A multitude of vitamins, minerals, phytonutrients, and healthy fats are proving to be essential as a defense against skin cancer and as protective agents for overall skin health. It's almost impossible to single out one SuperFood or SuperNutrient that is best for skin health. In fact, it's probably the effects of nutrient synergy that offer benefits beyond what each nutrient can offer individually.

That said, the SuperNutrients and SuperFoods that follow have been shown to be particularly beneficial for the health of your skin.

Vitamin C

Recommended amount: Supplemental vitamin C for skin health (or any other reason) should not exceed 2000 milligrams a day, taken in divided doses, which means you should take 250 to 500 milligrams up to four times a day. This is in addition to dietary sources of vitamin C. Aim for at least 350 milligrams a day from a combination of the following foods (there is no upper limit to the amount of dietary vitamin C you can safely eat in a day):

1 large yellow bell pepper = 341 mg
1 large red bell pepper = 312 mg
1 guava = 165 mg
1 large green bell pepper = 132 mg
1 cup fresh orange juice = 124 mg (97 mg a cup from frozen concentrate)
1 cup fresh strawberries = 97 mg
1 medium navel orange = 80 mg
1 cup fresh broccoli (chopped) = 79 mg
1 medium kiwi = 57 mg

Vitamin C is one of the most studied antioxidants in science. It is a prominent factor in reducing inflammation, which, as in other organ systems, plays a role in skin health. It has been shown to help prevent heart disease and some forms of cancer, and high blood levels have been inversely associated with all-cause mortality. All antioxidants communicate with vitamin C in one way or another.

Vitamin C is naturally found in skin tissue. Once inside the skin, vitamin C helps neutralize free radicals that are formed by exposure to UV light. When the skin's supply of vitamin C is depleted—for example, through sun exposure, smoking, or pollution—the skin's ability to prevent and repair free radical damage is compromised. The end result for your face is sun damage, wrinkles, and spots of uneven hyperpigmentation (darkening of the skin). In a 2003 double-blind study to see if vitamin C could help lighten sun-damaged skin that had darkened unevenly over time, participants had topical vitamin C applied to half of the face and a placebo to the other side. The results showed a significant improvement of the vitamin C–treated side.

It turns out that vitamin C can also boost the production of collagen in the skin. Collagen is an essential protein that keeps your skin firm and toned. When collagen is not produced properly, your skin can begin to sag and will lose its vitality. Collagen is also an important element in the health of the connective tissue throughout your body.

Wound healing is also dependent on vitamin C. As we age we may have lower levels of skin vitamin C, which can mean that healing of wounds in the skin does not happen as well as it did when we were young.

No direct association has been made between the overall consumption of citrus fruits, which contain large amounts of vitamin C, and skin cancer. However, consumption of D-limonene, a flavonoid found in the peel of oranges, grapefruits, and lemons, has been associated with a decreased risk of squamous-cell cancer (SCC) of the skin. A second study also looked at the risk for SCC, but this time researchers added black tea to their study of limonene. They found that consumption of citrus peel, black tea, and both together were associated with a lower risk of squamous cell carcinoma. Interestingly, the group that consumed both black tea and citrus peel had a significantly lower risk of SCC than either the black tea or citrus peel groups individually, demonstrating once again that the synergy of phytonutrients increases beneficial effects.

Because of all the benefits vitamin C has for your skin, bringing this nutrient into your diet and skin-care regimen can help you look and feel better, reduce the look of wrinkles, and improve your skin's quality.

Vitamin E

Recommended amount: For supplemental vitamin E, I recommend 100 to 200 IU a day. If you take supplemental vitamin E, be sure it contains all eight forms, including four tocopherols and four tocotrienols, and ideally as much gamma tocopherol as alpha tocopherol. Some of my favorite brands are MaxiVision Whole Body Formula and SuperFoodsRx Daily Packettes. For tocotrienols, I recommend Kyäni Sunset Omega-3/ Tocotrienols (www.kyani.net). This is in addition to food sources of vitamin E. Aim for at least 16 milligrams a day from a combination of the following foods (although you can have as much dietary vitamin E as you like):

Best sources of alpha tocopherols:
2 tablespoons wheat germ oil = 41 mg (total tocopherols)
2 tablespoons canola oil = 13.6 mg
2 tablespoons peanut oil = 9.2 mg
1 ounce raw almonds (22–24 nuts) = 7.7 mg
¼ cup hulled dry-roasted sunflower seeds = 6.8 mg
2 tablespoons raw (untoasted) wheat germ = 5 mg
1 ounce hazelnuts (20 nuts) = 4.3 mg
1 medium orange bell pepper = 4.3 mg
2 tablespoons olive oil = 4 mg
2 tablespoons peanut butter = 3.2 mg
1 kiwi = 3 mg
1 cup blueberries (1 baseball) = 2.8 mg
2 tablespoons soybean oil = 2.6 mg
1 avocado = 2 mg

Best sources of gamma tocopherol (there are no recommended amounts):
Pistachios
Pecans
Walnuts
Pumpkin seeds
Cashews
Peanuts

Best sources of tocotrienols (there are no recommended amounts):

Oats
Oat bran
Rye
Wheat bran
Barley
Black olives
Macadamia nuts
Pistachios

When you hear the term "vitamin E," you may think it refers to one single substance. In reality, vitamin E refers to a family of fat-soluble vitamins that are active throughout the body. Four are called tocopherols and four are called tocotrienols, and all eight forms play a role in achieving SuperHealth. Vitamin E is a major antioxidant that protects fatty acids from damage by free radicals. Even then, vitamin E does not work alone. It's a team player that does its best work when accompanied by vitamin C, vitamin B_3, selenium, glutathione, polyphenols, and carotenoids.

Studies have shown that vitamin E, like vitamin C, may be helpful in reducing hyperpigmentation, and its antioxidant function may help in scavenging free radicals produced by UV radiation. Topical vitamin E has been shown to have a wide variety of skin benefits, including repairing rough, dry skin, decreasing the effects of psoriasis and erythema (redness of the skin due to overexposure to the sun), and possibly reducing the appearance of stretch marks on the skin.

Oral vitamin E supplementation for the skin should be a mixture of tocopherols and tocotrienols. Topical vitamin E creams or gels should be in the form of d-alpha-tocopherol and should be applied every morning.

VITAMIN A

Recommended amount: For supplemental vitamin A (in the form of retinol, or preformed vitamin A), take no more than 3000 IU per day. If you take more than that, you may increase your risk for bone fractures. For nonanimal food sources of vitamin A, aim for a combination of the following foods (there is no increased risk of fracture from carotenoid sources of vitamin A):

Alpha-carotene: Aim for 2.4 milligrams a day from a combination of the following foods:

1 cup canned pumpkin (1 baseball) = 11.7 mg
1 cup cooked carrots (slices) (1 baseball) = 6.6 mg
10 raw baby carrots = 3.8 mg
1 cup cooked butternut squash (cubes) (1 baseball) = 2.3 mg
1 large orange bell pepper (1 baseball) = .3 mg
1 cup cooked collard greens (chopped) (1 baseball) = .2 mg

Beta-carotene: Aim for 6 milligrams a day from a combination of the following foods:

1 cup cooked sweet potato (1 baseball) = 23 mg
1 cup canned pumpkin (1 baseball) = 17 mg
1 cup cooked carrots (sliced) (1 baseball) = 13 mg
1 cup cooked spinach (1 baseball) = 11.3 mg
1 cup cooked kale (chopped) (1 baseball) = 10.6 mg
1 cup cooked butternut squash (cubes) (1 baseball) = 9.4 mg
1 cup cooked collard greens (chopped) (1 baseball) = 9.2 mg

Beta-cryptoxanthin: Aim for 1 milligram per day from a combination of the following foods:

1 cup cooked butternut squash (cubes) (1 baseball) = 9.4 mg
1 cup cooked red bell pepper (strips) (1 baseball) = 2.8 mg
1 Japanese persimmon (2½ inches in diameter) = 2.4 mg
1 cup mashed papaya (1 baseball) = 1.8 mg

1 large red bell pepper (raw) (1 baseball) = .8 mg
1 cup fresh tangerine juice = .5 mg
1 medium tangerine (½ baseball) = .3 mg

Vitamin A, which is also known as retinol, is perhaps the most important oral and topical vitamin for the appearance of the skin. It is one of the few substances with a molecular structure small enough to penetrate the outer layers of the skin, which then allows it to help repair the lower layers where collagen and elastin are found. Retinol has been shown to stimulate new collagen production, which means that it works to diminish wrinkles and fine lines. It also works to help lighten the brown spots that appear with age.

Due to the reduced production of collagen as we age, the skin becomes thinner and rougher. Vitamin A can help reverse those conditions, according to a 2004 study that treated participants with a retinol lotion three times a week for twenty-four weeks. The results showed that retinol increased the production of glycosaminoglycan and procollagen, two structural components of the skin—and wrinkles, roughness, and overall aging severity were all significantly reduced. The authors concluded that because of the production of those two compounds, retinol-treated skin "is more likely to withstand skin injury and ulcer formation along with improved appearance."

There are two general categories of vitamin A, depending on whether the food source is an animal or a plant. Vitamin A found in foods that come from animals is called preformed vitamin A. It is absorbed in the form of retinol, one of the most usable (active) forms of vitamin A. Sources include egg yolks, fortified dairy, Smart Balance buttery spread, and a multivitamin. There are three carotenoids from plants that your body can convert to vitamin A: beta-carotene, alpha-carotene, and beta-cryptoxanthin.

PROTECTION FROM SKIN CANCER

One of the most important reasons for following this week's SuperHealth recommendations is to help reduce your risk of skin cancer. The foods and nutrients in this chapter all have, to one degree or another, the ability to protect against sun damage, which not only visibly ages your skin but is the leading cause of skin cancer.

Skin cancer is the most common of all cancers; it accounts for almost half of all cancers in the United States. The American Cancer Society estimated about 60,000 new cases of melanoma (a form of skin cancer that arises in melanocytes, the cells that produce pigment; it is curable if diagnosed early but sometimes can be fatal) were diagnosed in the United States in 2007, resulting in more than eight thousand deaths. More than 1 million cases of non-melanoma skin cancer are found in this country each year.

If you're younger than age sixty and diagnosed with skin cancer, your risk for multiple systemic cancers is significantly increased. Therefore, healthy skin equals healthy immune system equals decreased risk not only for skin cancer, but also for systemic cancers like breast cancer, prostate cancer, non-Hodgkin's lymphoma, and leukemia.

There has been a dramatic increase in all types of skin cancer in the past two decades. There probably are a number of reasons for this, but the most significant risk factor for skin cancer is increased exposure to ultraviolet (UV) light from the sun and from tanning beds. UV rays cause damage to cell membranes and DNA, leading to DNA strand breaks and eventual mutations. It is difficult to explain to a tan-obsessed society, especially to teens and young adults who consider themselves immortal, that what looks good now can kill you later on.

Although you do want to get about fifteen to twenty minutes of sunlight exposure without sunscreen three to four times a week to be sure you're getting enough vitamin D, you don't want to tan or burn. In addition to the usual advice of avoiding the sun between 10:00 a.m. and 3:00 p.m. (if your shadow is shorter than you are, the sun's rays are at their strongest), be sure to use sunscreen that's at least SPF 15 or higher. Choose a "sport" version that stays on in the water, put it on about twenty minutes before you go out into the sun, and reapply it every couple of hours.

Don't forget to put sunscreen on your face, especially your nose, ears, and even your lips (or use a lip balm that has an SPF factor of 15 or higher). These are the places where the most dangerous skin cancers are likely to form, so you want to protect them as much as possible.

For the complete Week 5 Planner, see page 310.

My Personal Tanning Secret

The best "natural tan" I know is to drink one cup of organic carrot juice daily, as well as one cup of R.W. Knudsen Very Veggie Vegetable Cocktail (low sodium). Drink them about six to eight hours apart to prevent competition between the carotenoids for bioavailability. If you don't like carrot juice (and I didn't when I first started drinking it), start off with ¼ cup, then go to ½ cup, then to a full cup. You'll find that you actually enjoy the taste after a short while—I know I do. Along with the two juices, add a SuperHealth Spinach Salad (see page 280) three to four times a week, be patient, and within four to eight weeks the color from these carotenoids will be in your skin.

◆ MEET LINA MILLARD ◆

Walking Her Way to Health

Eighty-two-year-old Lina Millard first came out to California from the Midwest during World War II to help her sister who was having a baby. She got a job as a riveter working for Convair on B-24s. She liked California so much that she moved there with her whole family.

She got married and raised a family of seven children. When her husband died, her oldest was fifteen and her youngest was a year and a half. It was her seven children who kept her going, and kept her busy. But one thing she always found time for was walking.

"When I was pregnant with my first child," says Millard, "the doctor told me I should be walking. So I made it a point to get out and walk, and I never stopped. In earlier years I would walk two or three miles with a friend. These days I still walk with a friend, but we walk for about an hour, six days a week."

Besides the walking, Millard says she has always eaten healthfully, although since seeing Dr. Pratt for some eye problems, she's added a lot more spinach and fish and green leafy vegetables to her diet. She says she does have a few "secrets" about how she's lived so well into her eighties.

"I don't get bored," she explains. "I keep busy. But when I relax, I totally relax. I learned early on that if I need a nap, I take one. When the kids were resting, I would nap—for a half hour at the most—but it was all I needed. I found that if I tried to work through it, I just kept getting slower and slower. So I got more done if I stopped for a nap first.

"I keep my mind active, too. I discuss politics with my grandchildren. I don't go to extremes—nobody has to agree with me. When they're old enough to vote, I tell them to make up their own minds. We may disagree, and we may vote differently, but we have a good time hashing it out first."

Millard also says she never lets life get her down. She may be walking a little less than she used to, but she's now gardening more, and that gives her exercise and keeps her spirits up. "I've been through a lot in my life," she says, "but I raised seven great kids and I now have nine terrific grandchildren. I have a lot to be thankful for as well."

8

Step 6: Preserve Your Senses

For your basics, see the SuperHealth Food Pyramid, page 19 (for your bonus see below)

Week 6 SuperFoods:

Pomegranates	Kiwis
Blueberries	Oranges
Walnuts	Wheat germ
Spinach	Almonds

When you get older, you want to be able to remember your birthday, count your candles, hear the conversations, the music, and the wonderful sounds of nature, and enjoy the guests at your party. That's what all the steps in the SuperHealth program are leading to—to be able to flame out at the finish line still being able to see, hear, smell, taste, feel, and think your way independently in the world. Following the six steps in this book not only adds years to your life; it gives you the best chance of preserving your senses as you mature, which makes the quality of those extra years far better than they might be otherwise.

The same powerful nutrients, antioxidants, and anti-inflammatories that keep your heart and lungs healthy, keep your blood sugar under control, and keep your blood circulating also help keep your eyesight, hearing, and brain sharp as you get older. And there is a direct relationship between the health of your senses and the health of your body. Studies have shown that people who have cataracts and macular degeneration also have a higher incidence of cardiovascular disease and premature death. So the obvious strategy is protect your senses, protect your life.

There's another important reason to preserve your senses, and that is because it allows you to stay in touch with the world. Socialization plays a large role in preserving good health as you get older. If you're homebound and you can't see, can't hear, can't communicate with the world, your total health picture is not going to be very positive. I always use my mother as a role model in that respect. She was a great socializer. Even when she eventually went to live in an assisted-living facility, she made it her business to get to know everyone there. She made friends wherever she went. If she couldn't get out, she used the telephone as her means of connection. She was as sharp as a tack until the end, and I know it was due to her energy and enthusiasm for remaining an active participant in the world around her.

As always, nutrition is the cornerstone of keeping your senses intact and your brain in tip-top shape. You've been introduced earlier to five of the eight SuperFoods in this chapter—blueberries, walnuts, spinach, oranges, and wheat germ—and you'll be reading about three for the first time—pomegranates, kiwis, and almonds. All of them have been included here because of particular nutrients they possess that help mitigate some of the age-related changes our brains and senses experience during the maturing process.

POMEGRANATES

Recommended amounts: ½ cup to 1 cup (4 to 8 ounces) of 100% pomegranate juice, five to seven days a week.

Pomegranates, which have been around since ancient

times, have long been recognized for their health benefits. Recent studies have shown that the consumption of pomegranate juice can lower blood pressure in hypertensive people (those with high blood pressure). We've all heard the warnings about keeping blood pressure in check for cardiovascular health, but it turns out that high blood pressure also puts you at risk for degenerative eye diseases and for decreased cognitive abilities. A long-term Finnish study tracked 1,450 middle-aged men and women for twenty-one years. Those with the highest blood pressure had twice the risk of Alzheimer's disease and dementia in later life. Pomegranate juice can be an effective part of your pressure-lowering regimen.

It also appears that pomegranate juice might be helpful in preventing certain types of hearing loss, as it has been found to stimulate vasodilation (widening of the blood vessels, which leads to increased blood flow). Reduced blood flow to the cochlea (an important hearing center) appears to play a role in hearing loss, as it does in age-related macular degeneration (AMD). There is reduced blood flow to the eye in AMD patients compared to people of the same age who do not have AMD. Cellular metabolism clearly depends on adequate oxygen and nutrients as well as the proper elimination of waste products. If the blood flow to an organ system is good, you usually find that organ system is in good health. Pomegranates are also phytochemical powerhouses—they have two to three times the antioxidant power of green tea or red wine and also possess potent anti-inflammatory chemicals, which is one reason they have been shown to reduce the risk of cardiovascular disease and cancer.

Many people shy away from the pomegranate because it is a difficult fruit to eat. However, you can get the benefits of the fruit without any mess or fuss by drinking pomegranate juice such as Pom Wonderful 100% Pomegranate Juice (which can be found in most supermarkets or at www.pomwonderful.com) and R.W. Knudsen 100% Pomegranate Juice. If you find the taste of pomegranate juice somewhat bitter, you can try combination juices such as pomegranate-blueberry juice, pomegranate-cherry juice, or pomegranate-cranberry juice. One of my favorite blends is Trader Joe's Triple Berry Juice, which is a 100% juice blend of pomegranate, blueberry, and cranberry. Avoid brands that contain added sugar. You can use the juice in sauces, vinaigrettes, and marinades, but the best way to enjoy it is to mix it with seltzer and a slice of lemon or lime.

Blueberries

Recommended amount: 1 to 2 cups (1 to 2 baseballs) daily

Sidekicks: purple grapes, cranberries, boysenberries, raspberries, strawberries, fresh currants, blackberries, cherries, goji berries, açai berries, lingonberries, and all other varieties of fresh, frozen, or freeze-dried berries

Berries are good for the brain. Researchers have found that blueberries can help to protect the brain against oxidative stress and inflammation, both of which play important roles in brain aging. Both inflammatory markers and cellular and molecular oxidative damage increase during normal brain aging. But studies have shown that consumption of a diet rich in antioxidant and anti-inflammatory agents such as those found in blueberries and their sidekicks may lower the risk of developing age-related neurodegenerative diseases such as Parkinson's disease and Alzheimer's disease.

Animal studies have shown that blueberry extracts improve memory, and in rats whose genes produce the beta-amyloid-rich plaques found in Alzheimer's disease, blueberries make the rats perform better in maze tests even though the rats still get the plaques. It seems that in most species studied, including humans, the appearance of plaque does not always mean clinical disease is present or inevitable.

In another study blueberry supplementation given to rats equal to one cup daily in humans for two months has been shown to improve the motor functions of balance, coordination, and memory. Dr. James A. Joseph of the Human Nutrition Research Center on Aging at

Tufts University has conducted a number of studies about our little berry friends, and he reports that blueberries, blackberries, cranberries, Concord grape juice, and strawberries have been effective in reversing motor behavior deficits (all in lab rats so far—let's hope we can all be "rat-like" in this regard).

Blueberries are delicious mixed into a bowl of yogurt, topped with a sprinkle of wheat germ, and spiced with cinnamon. And while they were once a seasonal fruit, frozen blueberries (and most other berries as well) are now readily available all year long. I always keep some in my freezer and put a cup or so of frozen berries in a container in the refrigerator to defrost overnight so I can sprinkle them into my cereal or yogurt in the morning. You can add berries while still frozen to pancakes, muffins, and quick-bread batter. And for a quick summer snack, nothing beats a cup or two of frozen purple grapes to cool down a hot day.

Walnuts

Recommended amount: 1 handful (1 layer on your palm), five times a week

Sidekicks: almonds, pistachios, sesame seeds, peanuts, pumpkin and sunflower seeds, macadamia nuts, pecans, hazelnuts, cashews

Walnuts have often been thought of as a "brain food," not only because of the wrinkled brainlike appearance of their shells but also because of their high concentration of omega-3 fats. Our brains are made up of more than 60 percent fat, so they rely on a steady supply of good fats—like the omega-3s found in walnuts—to promote the varied activities of the brain. The membranes of all our cells, including our brain cells or neurons, are primarily composed of fats. Anything that wants to get into or out of a cell must pass through the cell's outer membrane. And omega-3 fats, which are especially fluid and flexible, make this process a whole lot easier, maximizing the cell's ability to usher in nutrients while eliminating wastes.

There is also a link between walnuts and the health

of your eyes. A study published in the *Archives of Ophthalmology* found that these tasty nuts can help prevent the progression of age-related macular degeneration (AMD). Researchers found that while high intake of animal fat increased AMD and processed foods doubled the risk of AMD, patients who ate more than one serving of nuts a week decreased their risk of AMD progression by more than 50 percent.

In addition, walnuts contain melatonin, an important immune system booster, as well as an antioxidant compound called ellagic acid that supports the immune system and appears to have several anticancer properties. Walnuts also contain alpha-linolenic acid (ALA), an essential omega-3 fatty acid, and other polyphenols that act as antioxidants and may block the adverse cellular signals resulting from free radical exposure that can later produce compounds that would increase inflammation.

Spinach

Recommended amount: 1 cup steamed (1 baseball) or 2 cups raw, five to seven days a week

Sidekicks: kale, collard greens, Swiss chard, arugula, mustard greens, turnip greens, bok choy, romaine lettuce, seaweed, purslane

As we know, carotenoids, including alpha-carotene and beta-carotene, lutein, lycopene, zeaxanthin, and beta-cryptoxanthin, which produce the red, yellow, and orange colors found in many fruits and vegetables, are antioxidants that help to act as anti-inflammatories, preserve our muscles, protect our brain, strengthen the immune system, reduce the risk of various types of cancer, reduce the risk of type 2 diabetes, help reduce the risk of arthritis, and play a significant role in preventing cardiovascular disease. Now we find another role for these free radical fighters: They help reduce the risk of cataracts and macular degeneration.

In particular, we find that lutein and zeaxanthin, found in spinach and its sidekick, green leafy vegetables, offer a powerful reduction of the risk of these ailments. One study that showed this to be the case is the Nurses' Health Study, which followed 50,461 women between the ages of forty-five and seventy-one for up to twelve years. The results showed that the carotenoids lutein and zeaxanthin were the greatest deterrents to cataracts, and that participants who consumed either raw or cooked spinach at least twice a week lowered their risk by 30 to 38 percent as compared to those who consumed spinach less than once a month.

The macula (the part of the retina that gives us our 20/20 vision) contains the highest accumulation of lutein and zeaxanthin in the body. Macular pigment filters blue light, which is particularly damaging to the eye. Lutein and zeaxanthin absorb blue light (a specific damaging wavelength of light), thereby helping in the filtering process. Lutein and zeaxanthin are also both powerful antioxidants and protect the retina from free radical damage, which can promote the onset of macular degeneration.

Spinach is also an excellent brain food. In animal studies, researchers have found that spinach may help protect the brain from oxidative stress and may reduce the effects of age-related declines in brain function. Researchers found that feeding aging laboratory animals spinach-rich diets significantly improved both their learning capacity and their motor skills.

Multivitamins for Your Eyes

For general eye health, my recommendation is to take a multivitamin that contains at least the following: lutein, zeaxanthin, alpha-lipoic acid, zinc with copper, vitamin C, and a full spectrum of vitamin E. A good choice is Maxivision Whole Body Formula, or the SuperFoodsRx Daily Dose Packettes (www.superfoodsrx.com) plus 6 milligrams of supplemental lutein (such as Carlson Lutein, www.carlsonlabs.com). This supplement should be combined with an EPA/DHA supplement (500 to 1000 milligrams a day for adult women and 1000 to 2000 milligrams for adult men).

Kiwis

Recommended amount: multiple times a week
Sidekicks: Brazilian pineapple, and strawberry guava

Spinach isn't the only food that's good for your eyes. It turns out that kiwis are an excellent nonleafy green source of lutein and zeaxanthin, which have been found to be protective against cataracts and macular degeneration.

Kiwis are also an excellent source of vitamin C. This nutrient is the primary water-soluble antioxidant in the body, neutralizing free radicals that can cause damage to cells and lead to problems such as inflammation and cancer. In fact, adequate intake of vitamin C has been shown to be an immune system booster and is helpful in reducing the severity of conditions like osteoarthritis, rheumatoid arthritis, and asthma, and for preventing conditions such as colon cancer, atherosclerosis, and diabetic heart disease. Kiwis are also a good source of the important fat-soluble antioxidant vitamin E. Both vitamins C and E are excellent for brain, eye, and hearing health, and kiwis give you both. Kiwis are available in most supermarkets all year round. The most common variety is Hayward, which has green flesh and is covered with brown fuzz. Rub off the fuzz and you can actually eat the whole kiwi, skin and all. Slice kiwis over your morning cereal or lunchtime yogurt, add chunks of kiwi to turkey or tuna salads, or puree kiwis in your smoothies.

Oranges

Recommended amount: 1 medium orange (1 baseball); ½ cup orange juice daily
Sidekicks: lemons, white and pink grapefruits, kumquats, tangerines, limes

We already know about the high concentrations of vitamin C and polyphenols in oranges. But oranges are also naturally rich in folate, or folic acid, a B vitamin. One role of folate is to help our bodies process the amino acid homocysteine, which in high levels seems to promote the buildup of fatty plaques in the blood vessels (atherosclerosis) and promotes inflammation. High homocysteine has also been associated with increased risk for macular degeneration and cardiovascular disease, and it may be associated with twice the risk of dementia and Alzheimer's disease. Vitamins B_6 and B_{12} and folic acid work together to effectively control homocysteine levels, which also influence oxidative stress. When folate is lacking, homocysteine is not broken down; it builds up in our bodies and promotes inflammation, leading to an increased risk for ailments like cardiovascular disease, degenerative eye disease, and Alzheimer's disease.

Another phytonutrient oranges contain is the flavonene hesperidin. In animal studies hesperidin has been shown to lower high blood pressure and cholesterol and also to have strong anti-inflammatory properties. This component is found in the peel and inner white pulp of the orange, so to reap the full benefits of oranges, grate a tablespoon of the peel and use it to flavor tea, salads, yogurt, soups, and cereals, or just rinse the peel off with tap water and take a bite of it.

More About Homocysteine

In addition to B_6, B_{12}, and folic acid, there are two more compounds that seem to be important in the fight against high homocysteine levels: betaine and choline. High homocysteine levels can come from a deficiency in B_6, B_{12}, folic acid, betaine, and choline, or you just may be genetically coded with the high homocysteine marker. The best sources of betaine are spinach, broccoli, and beets, while choline is found in eggs, cod, shrimp, navy beans, wild salmon, broccoli, Brussels sprouts, cauliflower, asparagus, spinach, green peas, and soybeans. Choline and betaine help to promote proper cell membrane function, assist in nerve-muscle communication, and prevent the buildup of homocysteine, which in high amounts is related to everything from macular degeneration to Alzheimer's disease to cardiovascular disease and stroke. In addition to getting your B_6, B_{12}, and folic acid from supplements, it's also very important to include dietary sources of choline and betaine that come from SuperFoods (see page 272 for the best sources of choline and betaine).

Wheat Germ

Recommended amount: 2 tablespoons a day (2 tablespoons = 1 shot glass)

Sidekick: Wheat-free oat bran (if you are on a gluten-free diet)

I grew up eating wheat germ. In fact, I remember my mother making me take a spoonful of wheat germ oil every day. It was not a pleasant thing to do—I would hold my nose and swallow it down. But, as usual, it turns out Mom knew what she was doing (although there's no need to take wheat germ oil—sprinkling wheat germ on a variety of foods works just as well). In addition to its role as a Super Whole Grain Sidekick, wheat germ stands on its own as one of the best sources of folic acid. It is also an excellent source of magnesium and vitamin E, which has been shown to help maintain cognitive function as we age. Vitamin E has also been linked with a host of health benefits including improving vitality, promoting a healthy heart, and strengthening the immune system, and magnesium is important in preventing cardiovascular disease, cellular aging, and diabetes.

Because of its unsaturated fat content, wheat germ goes rancid easily, especially if it's raw. Always store opened wheat germ in the refrigerator in a tightly sealed container, where it will keep for up to nine months. Unopened jars will keep on the shelf for about one year.

Wheat germ makes a nutritious and often undetectable addition to myriad dishes, including breads, pancakes, waffles, cookies, cereals, and milkshakes, and it can be added to yogurt or cold cereals or hot oatmeal.

Almonds

Recommended amount: 1 layer on your palm, five days a week (alternate nut choices with walnuts and other sidekicks—see page 191—so that daily total equals 1 ounce or a layer spread across the palm)

Almonds are another excellent source of vitamin E. A 2005 study published in the *Journal of the American Dietetic Association* confirmed that eating almonds significantly increased vitamin E levels in the blood and red blood cells and almonds also helped lower cholesterol levels. Vitamin E is a powerful antioxidant that defends your cells against damage on a daily basis and prevents artery-clogging oxidation of cholesterol. Eating a handful of almonds a day is a great way to get the vitamin E your body needs to stay healthy. They are a good source of calcium and polyphenols (found in the brown skin) as well.

Almonds may also slow the absorption of carbohydrates into the body, which means that they help to create a slower rise in blood sugar levels—and therefore help to keep insulin levels in check. Almonds also cause greater levels of satiety, that is, satisfaction or fullness from food. This may be due to their high fiber content, and this greater satiety leads to an overall satisfaction of hunger that can help with maintaining a healthy weight.

Choose either raw almonds or almonds that have been dry roasted rather than cooked in oil. Since almonds have a high fat content, it is important to store them properly in order to protect them from becoming rancid. Store shelled almonds in a tightly sealed container in a cool, dry place away from exposure to sunlight. Keeping them cold will further protect them from rancidity and prolong their freshness. Refrigerated almonds will keep for several months; in the freezer they will keep for up to a year.

Week 6: Preserve Your Senses Daily Food Planner

The chart below is an example of how you can add this week's foods to your SuperHealth program. It doesn't mean these are the only foods you should eat for the week; they are just suggestions for what to add into your daily diet. Feel free to mix and match foods and days to your heart's content.

	Food Suggestion	**Daily Servings**
Day 1	Pomegranate	½ cup (4 ounces) 100% juice
	Blueberries	1 cup (1 baseball)
	Walnuts	1 handful (1 layer on your palm)
	Spinach	2 cups raw (2 baseballs)
	Orange	1 medium (1 baseball)
	Wheat germ	2 tablespoons (1 shot glass)
Day 2	Strawberries	2 cups (2 baseballs)
	Almonds	1 handful (1 layer on your palm)
	Romaine lettuce	2 cups (2 baseballs)
	Kiwi	1 kiwi
	Orange juice	½ cup (4 ounces)
	Wheat germ	2 tablespoons (1 shot glass)
Day 3	Pomegranate	½ cup (4 ounces) 100% juice
	Cherries	1 cup (1 baseball)
	Pistachios	½ handful (1 layer on half of your palm)
	Kale	1 cup steamed (1 baseball)
	Pink grapefruit	½ grapefruit
	Wheat germ	2 tablespoons (1 shot glass)
	Almonds	½ handful (1 layer on half of your palm)
Day 4	Pomegranate	½ cup 100% juice
	Purple grapes	1 cup (1 baseball)
	Pumpkin seeds	1 handful (1 layer on your palm)
	Arugula	2 cups raw (2 baseballs)
	Kiwi	1 kiwi
	Lemon	½ cup lemon juice
Day 5	Blueberries	1 cup (1 baseball)

	Food Suggestion	Daily Servings
	Cashews	½ handful (1 layer on half of your palm)
	Turnip greens	1 cup steamed (1 baseball)
	Tangerine	2 tangerines
	Wheat germ	2 tablespoons (1 shot glass)
	Almonds	1 handful (1 layer on half of your palm)
Day 6	Pomegranate	½ cup (4 ounces) 100% juice
	Cran-raspberry juice	1 cup (8 ounces) juice
	Pecans	1 handful (1 layer on your palm)
	Spinach	2 cups raw (2 baseballs)
	Kiwi	1 kiwi
	Pink grapefruit	½ grapefruit
Day 7	Pomegranate	½ cup (4 ounces) 100% juice
	Açai-blueberry juice	½ cup (4 ounces) juice
	Peanuts	½ handful (1 layer on half of your palm)
	Orange	1 medium (1 baseball)
	Wheat germ	2 tablespoons (1 shot glass)
	Almonds	½ handful (1 layer on half of your palm)
	Spinach	2 cups raw (2 baseballs)

WEEK 6 EXERCISE PLAN

Throughout this book we've seen that exercise is good for your heart, your lungs, your waistline, your cells, your skin, your muscles, and your bones. It's pretty clear that exercise is good for every part and function of your body, which of course includes your senses and your brain. So continue the exercise portion of the SuperHealth program and remember that although this is the last of the six steps, it's really the beginning of your SuperHealth way of life. Keep building on these exercises by increasing the number of sets and reps at a slow and steady pace. Every time you get comfortable with what you're doing, ratchet it up a notch and do a few more, both weight and reps.

These exercise recommendations are minimums—you can, of course, do more if you choose. You don't want to overtrain, though; anything beyond ninety minutes can lead to fatigue and injury (unless you're playing a game like tennis or softball). And remember that several of these exercises can be done while you're doing something else, like driving or talking on the phone, so they don't take away huge chunks of your busy daily schedule.

- **Walk the Walk:** Increase your walking time to at least 30 minutes, five to six days a week, and try to take 100 steps per minute. If you counted your steps last week via your pedometer, increase your amount by 500 steps for this week. So if you started last week with 4,500 steps each day, your goal for this week is 5,000 steps each day. Your ultimate goal is 10,000 steps a day.
- **Dr. Steve's Power Stairs Workout:** Increase the number of times you walk up and down the stairs in your home or office. Try for two to four days of 15 minutes each this week and increase your speed until you are running up and down the stairs.
- **Heel to Fanny:** Stand on stairs or an elevated area (this can be done on a flat surface as well) and hold on to the railing or the wall keeping your knees together. The left leg remains straight. With your right leg beginning in a straight position, bring your right heel to your fanny. You may not be able to touch your fanny, but take it as far as you can and hold it there for 5 seconds, then let it down slowly. When you can comfortably do 3 sets of 20 with each leg, add 5-pound ankle weights, and increase weight as you get stronger. This builds strength in the hamstrings, those big muscles in the backs of the thighs. Do this three or four days a week.
- **Sit-up/Crunch:** Lie on your back with your knees bent and your feet flat on the floor in front of you. Lie on an exercise mat or carpet rather than a hard floor to prevent back strain. Your feet should be as

wide apart as your hips. Place your arms crossed on your chest and keep your chin pointing upward. Curl up and forward so that your head, neck, and shoulder blades lift off the floor. Pause for a count of two, then slowly lower your shoulder blades, neck, and head to the starting position. Increase to 5 sets of 30, three days a week.

- **Isometric Curl:** Hold on to the back of the steering wheel (while at a stop sign or signal) at the five o'clock and seven o'clock positions with your palms facing toward you and your arms bent. This can also be done by grabbing the edge of a desk or table, palms facing up, elbows at your sides, shoulders down. The idea is to attempt to bring your hands up toward your shoulders (you won't actually be able to do it—the point is to get the resistance). Hold the position for 10 to 20 seconds and repeat 25 times using both arms. This helps to tone the biceps and the front part of the shoulder muscles. For maximum benefit, vary the amount of arm bend slightly for each rep, as this strengthens the muscle at varying degrees of use. Make sure to keep your shoulders down and back. Do this two to four times a week.

- **Isometric Extension:** Again, this is a nonmovement form of strengthening. This time you're pushing against the steering wheel, desk, or any other immobile surface, with the heel of your hand and your fingers pointing down. Try to extend or straighten your arms, using your body weight to resist. Hold the position for 10 to 20 seconds and repeat using both arms. This helps to tone the triceps (back of the arm). Do this two to four times a week.

- **Tennis Ball Squeeze:** Keep a tennis ball or other type of ball, soft or hard, at your desk, in the car, or around the house. Squeeze at least 20 times a day (more if you want). Squeezing the ball and holding it for a count of 20 can actually help lower your blood pressure. It's a good one to do while you're on the phone during a stressful conversation—stress is a major source of inflammation.

- **Stand Up/Sit Down:** This is one you can do anywhere, as many times as you want. Simply get up from your chair (do not use a chair with wheels) without using your arms to push you up. Do not lean forward to get momentum; the object is to use your leg muscles. Then sit slowly all the way back down into the chair, focusing on your quads, the muscles at the fronts of your thighs. As your quad muscles get stronger, go down until you're almost but not quite sitting and then come back up. This is another good exercise to do while you're talking on the phone. Repeat as many times as you like.

- **Wall Sit:** If your legs are weak or the Stand Up/Sit Down exercise is hard on your knees, start off with a Wall Sit instead. Place your butt, back, and shoulders flat against the wall, with your feet about hip-distance apart about 1.5 feet away from the wall. Slide your back down the wall so your knees are bending. Go as low as you can go to start (the goal is to form a 90-degree angle with your bent knees—if you do it right, your body should look like it's sitting in an invisible chair). Hold this for a count of 5, and slide back up the wall. Repeat with your feet straight ahead, and again with your toes facing inward. As you get stronger, slide farther down the wall until your legs are at a 90-degree angle and you are holding for a count of 10. Repeat as many times as you like.

- **Steering Wheel Squeeze:** While parked or at a red light, grip the steering wheel so that your hands are horizontally across from each other (at the three o'clock and nine o'clock positions). Your elbows are out and your arms should be forming a "C" shape. Try to push your hands together against the steering wheel—imagine that you're trying to close the "C" shape of your arms into an "O" shape. Hold this for 5 to 10 seconds, then let go. Repeat 10 times. This is great for building forearms, biceps, and shoulder muscles. You can try it outside the car, too: Grab either side of the back of a chair and try to push your arms from a "C" into an "O." Do this two to four times a week.

- **Bicep Curl:** Stand with your feet about hip-width apart, as you hold a light weight in each hand in front of the thighs. Choose a weight that allows you to easily do 3 sets of 20 curls (you can also use cans of soup or vegetables if you don't have weights). Your grip should be underhand (palms facing upward). Squeeze your biceps and bend your arms, curling the weights up toward your shoulders. Keep your elbows stationary and at the sides of your body and bring the weight only as high as you can without moving your elbows. Slowly lower the weights, keeping a slight bend in the elbows at the bottom (don't lock the joints and try to keep tension on the muscle). If you can easily do 3 sets of 10, add 5 pounds of weight. Repeat for 3 sets of 10 reps, two to three times a week.

- **Tricep Extension:** From a standing position with your feet about hip-width apart, hold a light weight (or can) in your right hand. Bend forward so that your upper torso is perpendicular to the floor, keeping your right arm straight at your side. Bend and raise your elbow up toward the ceiling until your arm is at a right angle at your side, then extend your arm backward until it's straight. If you can easily do 2 sets of 10, add 2.5 to 5 pounds of weight, and increase in 2.5- to 5-pound increments. Repeat for 2 sets of 10, then repeat with your left arm. Do this two to four times a week.

- **Waist Twist:** Standing with your legs about shoulder-width apart, place a broom with a long handle or a dowel that's about six feet long behind your neck. Grasp the broom with both hands, palms facing forward. Start out with your entire body facing forward. then without moving the lower half of your body, twist from your waist as far as you can to your right. Go back to center, then twist as far as you can to your left. Repeat for 3 sets of 30 to 50, three to four days a week.

- **Side Bends:** Standing with your legs about shoulder-width apart, place a broom with a long handle or a dowel that's about six feet long behind your neck. Grasp the broom with both hands, palms facing forward. Start out with your entire body facing forward, then without moving the lower half of your body, bend at your waist as far as you can to your right so that one end of the dowel is facing the floor and the other is facing the ceiling. Go back to center, then bend as far as you can to your left. Repeat for 3 sets of 30 to 50, three to four days a week.

- **Bicycle:** Lie on your back on an exercise mat. Lift your legs up in the air, then bend your knees so that your calves are at a right angle to your thighs. Keep your arms on the floor at your sides to stabilize your body, then begin to "pedal" as if you were riding a bike. Bicycle for 1 minute, three to four times a week.

- **Platysma Rock:** Here's a good way to get rid of that "turkey neck" we all hate: The muscle that runs from your clavicle to your jaw and the skin around your mouth is the platysma muscle. Flex that muscle by keeping your head at its normal, upright position while using your face and neck muscles to pull your lower lip down away from your upper lip, exposing your lower teeth entirely. Try to make the corners of your lips point downward. You should be making an inverted smile or grimacing face that tenses the muscles in your neck. Hold this face for 5 seconds, and release. Repeat 10 times or more a day. This is something you can easily do in the car, at your desk, or while watching your favorite TV show.

This week, add these two exercises:
- **Push-ups:** Lie chest-down on an exercise mat or carpet with your hands at shoulder level, palms flat on the floor and slightly more than shoulder-width

apart, your feet together and parallel to each other. Keep your legs straight and your toes tucked under your feet or stay on your knees if you haven't yet developed sufficient upper-body strength. Straighten your arms as you push your body up off the floor, keeping your palms fixed at the same position and your body straight. Try not to bend or arch your upper or lower back as you push up. Exhale as your arms straighten out. Pause for a few seconds. Lower your body until your chest touches the floor. Bend your arms and keep your palms in fixed position, keeping your body straight and feet together. Try not to bend your back. If you can, keep your knees off the floor, and inhale as you bend your arms. Pause for a few seconds. Begin straightening your arms for a second push-up. Exhale as you raise your body. (If you don't have enough arm strength for push-ups on the floor, you can begin by leaning against a surface like the kitchen sink. Grasp the edge of the sink, palms facing away from you. Your upper body is touching the sink while you move your feet backward until your body is at a 20- 30-, or 45-degree angle. Your arms should be bent, elbows out. Keeping your body straight, push yourself slowly away from the sink until your arms are straight, pause for a few seconds, and move your chest back to touching the sink.) Start off with 3 sets of 5 and build up to 3 sets of 20. Do this two to three times a week.

If can't do push-ups this way because of injury or because you're still building up enough strength, there are a lot of other ways to do them that are less strenuous. For example, as mentioned above, you can do the push-ups on your knees instead of your feet, which lowers the amount of weight you're lifting. Or if you stand three to four feet away from a counter and place your palms on the edge of the counter, fingers up, shoulder-width apart, you can slowly lower yourself and do a half-push-up by bending your elbows and keeping your feet stationary.

- **Pull-ups:** Purchase a pull-up bar at any sporting

goods store and fasten it in a hallway or door frame. Grasp the bar with both hands, shoulder-width apart, palms facing away from you. Bend your knees so that your feet are off the floor. Pull yourself up with your arms until your chin is level with the bar. Your first goal is to be able to do 10 in a row. At that point, build up until you can do 3 sets of 10. Do this two to three times a week.

My final recommendation for the SuperHealth exercise program is to join a dance class, whether it's ballroom, swing, jazz, salsa, or hip-hop—it doesn't matter as long as it gets you moving. Dancing not only gives you aerobic exercise; it works all the basic muscle groups—and it's a great way to socialize as well.

Mom's Obstacle Course

There came a time in my mother's life when she couldn't see very well. But that didn't stop her from getting her exercise. What did she do? She set up her own obstacle course around the house. She'd walk a path around the living room to the dining room and into the kitchen, around the chairs and tables and then back again. She may not have been jogging for miles around the track, but she was getting the benefits of exercise nonetheless. If you can't get outside, you can do the same thing in your house. Set up your own obstacle course so that you have to walk to the right, walk to the left, climb over a few pillows, crawl under a chair . . . Make it fun and be like Mom—turn on the radio and have a blast. I have my own obstacle course I make up in the foothills near where I live. I go up and down hills, I jump over bushes, I duck under branches, I go around trees right and left. It may sound crazy, but I've done it for years. It keeps me alert and agile, and I love every minute of it.

Week 6: Preserve Your Senses Daily Exercise Planner

The chart below is an example of how you can add this week's exercises to your SuperHealth program. Now that you are at Week 6, ideally you should be doing thirty to ninety minutes of calorie-burning activity a day. The more time you can put in, the more benefits you will reap. And you don't have to do it all at once—you can fit many of these exercises into odd moments of your day. If you work at a sedentary job, take occasional ten-minute breaks and take a walk around the block or do some of the isometric exercises. At a minimum, try to do at least 80 percent of the exercises suggested below on any given day.

	Exercise	**Set Reminders**
Day 1	Walk	30 minutes
	Power Stairs	15 minutes; increase speed
	Heel to Fanny	3 sets of 20; add weight
	Isometric Curl	25 times with both arms; hold for 20 seconds
	Isometric Extension	25 times with both arms; hold for 20 seconds
	Ball Squeeze	20 times
	Steering Wheel Squeeze	3 sets of 20
	Waist Twist	3 sets of 30–50
	Side Bends	3 sets of 30–50
	Platysma Rock	20 times
	Push-ups	3 sets of 5
	Pull-ups	10 in a row
Day 2	Walk	30 minutes
	Heel to Fanny	3 sets of 20; add weight
	Sit-up/Crunch	5 sets of 30
	Isometric Curl	25 times with both arms; hold for 20 seconds
	Isometric Extension	25 times with both arms; hold for 20 seconds
	Bicep Curl	3 sets of 10; add weight
	Tricep Extension	3 sets of 10; add weight
	Bicycle	60 seconds

(continued)

	Exercise	Set Reminders
Day 3	Walk	30 minutes
	Power Stairs	15 minutes; increase speed
	Ball Squeeze	20 times
	Stand Up/Sit Down/Wall Sit	Unlimited times
	Steering Wheel Squeeze	3 sets of 20
	Waist Twist	3 sets of 30–50
	Side Bends	3 sets of 30–50
	Platysma Rock	20 times
	Push-ups	3 sets of 5
	Pull-ups	10 in a row
Day 4	Walk	30 minutes
	Heel to Fanny	3 sets of 20, add weight
	Sit-up/Crunch	5 sets of 30
	Isometric Curl	25 times with both arms; hold for 20 seconds
	Isometric Extension	25 times with both arms; hold for 20 seconds
	Ball Squeeze	20 times
	Stand Up/Sit Down/Wall Sit	Unlimited times
	Bicycle	60 seconds
Day 5	Walk	30 minutes
	Power Stairs	15 minutes; increase speed
	Isometric Curl	25 times with both arms; hold for 20 seconds
	Isometric Extension	25 times with both arms; hold for 20 seconds
	Ball Squeeze	20 times
	Bicep Curl	3 sets of 10; add weight
	Tricep Extension	3 sets of 10; add weight
	Waist Twist	3 sets of 30–50
	Side Bends	3 sets of 30–50
	Platysma Rock	20 times
Day 6	Walk	30 minutes
	Heel to Fanny	3 sets of 20; add weight
	Sit-up/Crunch	5 sets of 30
	Ball Squeeze	20 times
	Stand Up/Sit Down/Wall Sit	Unlimited times
	Steering Wheel Squeeze	3 sets of 20
	Bicycle	60 seconds

Exercise	Set Reminders
Push-ups	3 sets of 5
Pull-ups	10 in a row

Day 7	Walk	30 minutes
	Power Stairs	15 minutes; increase speed
	Isometric Curl	25 times with both arms; hold for 20 seconds
	Isometric Extension	25 times with both arms; hold for 20 seconds
	Bicep Curl	3 sets of 10; add weight
	Tricep Extension	3 sets of 10; add weight
	Waist Twist	3 sets of 30–50
	Side Bends	3 sets of 30–50
	Platysma Rock	20 times

EXERCISE, YOUR SENSES, AND YOUR BRAIN

Regular physical activity helps preserve adequate blood flow to all parts of the body. Physical activity also releases brain-derived neurotrophic factors (BDNFs—proteins that are responsible for the growth and survival of developing neurons) in the central nervous system. Too much loud noise can damage sensitive cells in the inner ear; however, several animal studies have shown that neurotrophic factors may prevent or reduce this inner-ear damage.

Exercise also plays a role in reducing the risk of age-related macular degeneration, a degenerative eye disease in which the light-sensitive cells in the back of the eye (the macula) stop working. There are two forms of AMD—wet and dry. Dry is the more common type, but it can lead to wet AMD. In wet AMD, there is a growth of abnormal blood vessels underneath the macula, and blood vessels leak into the retina. A 2006 study that followed almost four thousand people for fifteen years showed that those with an active lifestyle who exercised three or more times a week had a 70 percent lower risk of developing wet AMD; it also showed that those who regularly walked more than twelve blocks had a 30 percent lower risk of developing the disease.

If you need anything more to get motivated to start exercising, think about this: A 2001 study demonstrated that patients with Alzheimer's disease were less active (both intellectually and physically) in midlife and that this inactivity was associated with a *250 percent* increased risk of developing the disease. So if you're middle-aged and sitting around doing nothing, you might want to jog over to the newsstand to pick up a newspaper and a crossword puzzle book.

Once again, what's good for the heart is good for the brain. It turns out that aerobic exercise has important benefits for brain function because brain-derived neurotrophic factor (BDNF) is involved in the learning process, and it seems that aerobic exercise increases the production of BDNF. This is important because old brain cells die and new ones are generated throughout our lives, but the process slows down as we age. BDNF supports the survival of the existing cells.

An interesting study led by Arthur F. Kramer at the University of Illinois at Urbana-Champaign in 2006 involved a group of healthy but sedentary volunteers and put them into a six-month exercise program. Some did aerobic exercise—mostly walking—and some did toning exercises. By the end of the six-month program, the participants in the aerobic exercise group showed increases in brain volume compared with participants who did the toning and stretching exercises. The prefrontal and temporal parts of the brain—areas that show considerable age-related deterioration—incurred the greatest gains from aerobic exercise. Dr. Kramer told the news bureau of the university: "Moderate levels of exercise—in particular, walking—are relatively easy to do and may result in increased cognitive flexibility and the ability to lead independent lives for longer periods of time." In this case people who had been couch potatoes started with fifteen minutes of exercise, built it up to forty-five minutes, and subsequently showed improvements in brain volume and physical fitness.

In the well-respected Nurses' Health Study, which followed more than 18,000 women ages seventy to eighty-one for more than three decades, women who were the most physically active scored highest on tests of mental performance and had a 20 percent lower risk of mental impairment than women who were the least active. In this study physical activity did not have to be strenuous. Women who walked at a leisurely pace for at least six hours a week saw cognitive benefit, as did those who walked just two to three hours a week. This benefit is comparable to a three-year age difference. The message is clear: If you don't exercise, you'll have a brain that's older than your age. So just give yourself three hours of walking a week and you give yourself three years of better brain power!

Of course it's not only women who benefit. In a study of both men and women sixty-five and older, those who engaged in three or more hours of physical activity a week were 61 percent less likely than people not exercising to experience significant cognitive decline after two years.

MENTAL AEROBICS

More Lessons from Mom

My mom memorized phone numbers out of the phone book every morning and then checked her memory every afternoon to be sure she didn't lose her ability to remember things. She also listened to all the talk radio shows and daily news reports (she lost her reading vision with age-related macular degeneration in her eighties). She would talk with her kids, or anyone else who would listen, about current affairs on a daily or weekly basis. She played bridge all her life, and she played checkers with me all the time. Her memory was as sharp as could be up until her death at age ninety-one; her death certificate listed cause of death as "old age." And a lesson from Dad—he was a great one for chess; he made us kids play chess with him whenever he could catch us. He was also a reservoir of jokes. One year when I went back to medical school, we drove from Laguna Beach to Philadelphia. It took us a week. He told me at least one joke every hour for the entire trip. He could look at anything and say, "Oh, that reminds me of a joke," and off he'd go. He never ran out of material. It was good mental stimulation, and laughter boosts your immune system, so both of us had a fun and healthy trip.

We all know what happens to couch potatoes: They get fat and lazy. The brain responds the same way. Without mental exercise the brain goes off duty. In fact, in the late 1990s scientists discovered the first strong evidence that intellectual stimulation can significantly increase the number of brain cells in a crucial region of the mind. Activities such as playing card games, learning a musical instrument, and doing crossword puzzles or sudoku can keep the mind active. Here are some simple suggestions for exercising your brain:

- **Work your memory.** You may not want to memorize phone numbers, but memorization is good exercise for the brain. Try learning a new poem or, if it suits you, a prayer, every couple of days. It doesn't have to be particularly long; try to learn it in the morning and then recite it by heart in the evening.
- **Become a storyteller.** I often think about my grandfather, who was an excellent teller of tales. I couldn't wait to go to his house to spend the night because I knew I'd get an evening of great entertainment. If you have young children or grandchildren, have storytelling sessions where one person starts a story, the next person has to pick it up in the middle, then the next person picks it up from there, then back to the original storyteller. The sto-

ries can get hysterically funny. Kids love it and it's great mental exercise.

- **Play Ping-Pong.** Or tennis. Or any game that involves hand-eye coordination. The more neural circuits you light up, the greater the potential benefit. When you see the ball coming at you, the message is relayed to your brain and is then relayed to your muscles, which then move your arm and hand—so there is a lot going on in your brain before the movement takes place.

- **Become an expert.** The subject matter of your expertise doesn't really matter. Find a subject you're interested in and learn everything you can possibly discover about it. My mom became an expert in foreign and current affairs. She was a news junkie and couldn't wait to share and/or debate her ideas with her friends and family. She not only exercised her brain by filling it with all this information; she practiced socialization when she shared it with us all.

- **Be a mentor.** Even if you're not an expert in a particular subject, there are many ways you can mentor people younger than yourself. You probably have business or life experience that can be very useful and enlightening to those who may be just starting out in a career or simply need a few words of wisdom, or even just someone who will listen to them. It's great exercise for your brain, because when the person you are mentoring asks questions it causes you to think carefully in order to provide the best guidance and advice.

- **Walk to wake up your brain.** How many times have you considered one activity or another but talked yourself out of it with the old "I'm just so tired" excuse? Oftentimes it's not that we're so physically tired; it's that we're mentally fatigued. Fortunately, a new study has shown that low-intensity exercise—including walking—can be just what you need to perk up a sleepy mind. About 25 percent of the general population experiences mental fatigue at one time or another. Research has shown that instead of using caffeine and energy drinks to revive yourself, engaging in regular low-intensity exercise (such as walking, housework, washing the car, or pruning the bushes) can increase energy levels by 20 percent and decrease fatigue by 65 percent.

In the last ten to fifteen years more than ten studies have looked at self-reported mentally stimulating activities, and all but one of them found that older people who report being more intellectually active have a decreased risk of cognitive decline. Studies also find that those with the most education have better memory in their seventies—the more education, the better the memory. That sounds like a good reason to continue in school if you're there or to go back if you're not. Giving your brain a workout can make a difference.

KEEP YOUR SOCIAL CONNECTIONS

Here's another reason to get up off the couch and do something, preferably with other people: Socially isolated people have a two to four times increased risk of death of all causes compared to those with extended ties to friends, relatives, and the community in which they live. People attending cultural events, reading books or periodicals, playing music, or singing in a choir survived longer than nonparticipants of such activities in both Swedish and U.S. studies, and the beneficial effects were similar to and independent of the level of physical activity. This suggests that mechanisms other than increased cardiopulmonary fitness might be involved. Similar survival benefits have also been seen in people engaging in solitary activity such as reading books and newspapers or solving crossword puzzles (although these are solitary activities, there is still some engagement involved).

People who are engaged in life not only live longer; they live better. A February 2007 study in *Archives of*

General Psychiatry recruited 823 people (average age eighty-three) who did not have dementia and then studied the relationship between loneliness and Alzheimer's disease over four years: Those with the highest loneliness score had twice the risk for Alzheimer's as those with the lowest score. People who feel connected to others are more likely to thrive than those who are socially isolated. In fact, a major public health study involving more than 116,000 participants found that those who maintained a network of friends and family and pursued activities such as volunteering for community projects, had regular "game nights" with friends, or took a class had less mental decline and lived more active, pain-free lives.

Easing the Burden

Dr. John Rowe, chairman of the University of Connecticut Board of Trustees and former president of Mount Sinai NYU Health, told the *Harvard Public Health Review* in 2000 that we have enough data on how to maintain physical and cognitive function, reduce the risk for disease, and maintain productivity into old age so that aging populations do not have to become a staggering burden for society. "But," said Rowe, "it's not enough to add years of life. To make longevity meaningful in our culture, we must learn to integrate the wisdom and contributions of older Americans. We must develop a society that provides individuals with opportunities of continuing engagement in life. That is the final step of longevity."

TOP TIPS FOR PRESERVING THE SENSES

The wonderful thing about the SuperHealth program is that everything is interconnected. All the diet and lifestyle tips you've followed throughout the book are not only keeping you from dying prematurely; they're keeping you from aging prematurely. And that goes especially for your senses. There are, however, a few more steps you can take to be sure you give yourself the greatest likelihood of maintaining optimal hearing, eyesight, and cognitive functions throughout your life.

Avoiding Hearing Loss

According to the Better Hearing Institute, noise is one of the most common causes of hearing loss. The World Health Association estimates that 278 million people worldwide have moderate to severe hearing loss in one or both ears. Approximately 10 million Americans have already suffered irreversible hearing damage from noise, and another 30 million are exposed to dangerous noise levels every day. Excessive noise damages the hair cells in the organ of Corti within the cochlea, which are responsible for hearing high-frequency sounds. Over time and with continued exposure, both high and low tones are lost. Hearing loss related to hair-cell loss is not reversible and cannot be restored by a hearing aid.

Noise-induced hearing loss (NIHL) is a significant cause of disability and a major cost to society. Dangerous noise levels in the workplace are the most prevalent occupational hazard in the United States, and it can be exacerbated by noise in the environment like that from leaf blowers, lawn mowers, music players, and power tools.

Of course, noise is everywhere. Most of us don't even realize when the decibel levels of noise (the main unit of measurement for the loudness of a sound) are putting us at risk for hearing damage. To give you a better idea of how to compare decibel levels, here are some examples from the American Tinnitus Association:

Decibel Level (dB) Response	Source	Typical Physical
0	Softest sound that can be heard	None
10	Normal breathing	Barely audible
30	Whisper	Very quiet

Decibel Level (dB) Response	Source	Typical Physical
50–65	Normal conversation	Quiet
80–85	City traffic noise	Annoying
95–110	Motorcycle	Very annoying
100	School dance; boom box	Very annoying
105	Jackhammer	Risk of hearing damage after 1 hour
120	Nightclub	Can damage hearing after 15 minutes exposure per day (or night)
110–125	Stereo; personal music player	Can damage hearing after 15 minutes exposure per day
110–140	Rock concert; gunshot	Noise may cause pain and brief exposure can injure ears
150	Firecracker	Noise can cause pain and brief exposure can injure ears

SOUND PRESSURE LEVELS THAT CAN IRREVERSIBLY DAMAGE HEARING

dB	Duration	Sound Source	Industry
140	<1min	Firearms, jet engine	Military, aviation
130	>1min	Drop forge, jackhammers	Manufacturing, mines, construction
120	>5min	Amplified speakers	Musicians, recreational
110	>15min	Engines	Rail, trucking
100	>1hr	Woodshop, chainsaws	Forestry
90	>4hr	Motorcycles, lawn mowers	Recreational
85	>8h	Interior plane cabins	Aviation

10 Ways to Preserve Your Hearing

1. Wear hearing protection when noise levels are indicative of possible noise-induced hearing loss. You can use foam or silicone earplugs or muffs. Foam plugs are available at most pharmacies, while muffs and specialized ear protection can be found at sporting goods or electronics stores. The consistent use of hearing protection devices is the most important behavioral change you can make to prevent noise-induced hearing loss. Failure to use hearing protection for just thirty minutes during the workday in a loud-noise atmosphere reduces the protective device's effectiveness by 50 percent. There's also the group H.E.A.R.—Hearing Education and Awareness for Rockers (www.hearnet.com)—which makes custom earplugs for those who don't want to change the quality of what they're hearing as earplugs can do. They turn the volume down but have special filters that keep the spectrum true.

2. If you smoke, stop, and avoid secondhand smoke; this is a preventable risk factor for hearing loss. One study including more than three thousand people showed that smokers are nearly 70 percent more likely than nonsmokers to suffer hearing loss. The study found that passive smoking may increase the risk of becoming hearing impaired as well. Nonsmokers living with a smoker were found to be 1.94 times more likely to suffer from hearing problems than those who were not living with a smoker.

3. Take 250 milligrams of magnesium daily (in addition to the magnesium in your daily multivitamin). Zinc, folic acid, and vitamin B_{12} have also been shown to offer some protection against noise-induced hearing loss, so take a multivitamin such as Maxivison Whole Body Formula or the SuperFoods Rx daily supplement (SFRx Daily Dose).

4. Load up on SuperFoods, as high intake of dietary antioxidants can provide some protection.

5. Engage in physical activity—thirty to ninety minutes most days has been shown to be protective.

6. Supplement with magnesium, resveratrol, alphalipoic acid, N-acetylcysteine, and vitamin E, and eat ample protein—they all boost glutathione (the number one antioxidant in our cells) production, so taking the SFRx Cell Defense Supplement (in addition to your daily multivitamin) along with an early-morning serving of protein (aim for 5 to 10 grams of protein soon after waking up) will help glutathione levels in your cells. Some sample protein sources: 1 cup soymilk = 7 grams; 1 cup nonfat milk = 8 grams; 1 cup nonfat yogurt = 6 to 10 grams; 1 slice of Julian Bakery complete protein bread = 12 grams; 1 cup Kashi Go Lean High Protein and High Fiber Cereal = 13 grams.

7. Check with your health-care professional if you are taking certain types of drugs, including aminoglycosides, quinine, beta blockers, diuretics, nonsteroidal anti-inflammatory agents, salicylates, and tricyclic antidepressants, as these drugs are potentially ototoxic (harmful to hearing), especially if you are age sixty-five or older.

8. Purchase iPods or MP3 players that have a volume-level regulation feature, or turn down the volume. Consumer alert: We need MP3 players with decibel levels on the volume control and a warning light when harmful volumes are reached, and perhaps even a sound limit on the player itself.

9. Increase blood flow to the cochlea (where noise is processed and sent to the brain). Foods that have been shown to increase blood flow include purple grape juice (4 to 8 ounces a day), dark chocolate (100 calories a day), green or black tea (4 cups a day), pomegranate juice (4 to 8 ounces a day), berries (1 to 2 cups a day), and soy (10 to 15 grams soy protein a day). Aim for blood pressure readings of less than 115/80 (high blood pressure decreases blood flow), and don't forget physical activity.

10. Get a baseline hearing test (an initial test that determines if you have any hearing loss). All subsequent hearing tests will be measured against this first test, so you will know if your hearing has stayed the same or has gotten worse.

11 Ways to Prevent Cataracts and Age-Related Macular Degeneration

We often take our senses for granted, especially if they've served us well over the years. But our senses give us information about the world in which we live, and when our senses decline, our sense of the world changes as well. This can have a tremendous impact on your enjoyment of life, your social interactions, your ability to communicate, and your ability to be mobile in your environment.

What happens, for instance, when your sight begins to slowly diminish? It can mean a lot more than the annoyance of having to have a pair of reading glasses in every room or carrying a magnifying glass around with you. Vision loss can lead to everything from social isolation to falls, loss of driving privileges, and serious injury. That's why it's so important to preserve and maintain the health of our eyes. Here are eleven ways to help you do that:

1. While in the sun, wear a hat with a brim and wear sunglasses (wrapped) that block 100 percent of UVA/UVB and as much blue light as allowed by regulatory agencies. The Callaway golf company sunglass line meets these criteria.
2. Enjoy green leafy vegetables daily. Spinach, Swiss chard, and kale are three of the best. One serving equals 2 cups raw or ½ cup to 1 cup cooked. Aim for 12 milligrams a day of lutein from food (see page 259).
3. Enjoy a zeaxanthin-rich food daily. Aim for 3 milligrams a day in a combination of supplements and food. For instance:

- 1 large orange bell pepper
  8 mg
- approximately 50 goji berries (dried)
  1.5 mg
- 1 cup canned sweet yellow corn
  .9 mg
- 1 raw Japanese persimmon
  .8 mg
- 3.5 ounces wild Alaskan sockeye salmon (deck
  of cards)
  .75 mg
- 1 cup degermed cornmeal (baseball)
  .7 mg

4. Have two to four servings (3 to 4 ounces, or the size of a deck of cards) of wild Alaskan salmon (or sidekicks) per week.

5. Keep your BMI and waist circumference within the normal range (see page 340 for BMI and waist circumference charts).

6. Include thirty to ninety minutes of physical activity five times a week.

7. Have a handful of nuts (1 layer on the palm of your hand) five times a week. Walnuts, almonds, and pistachios should be part of your weekly mix.

8. Enjoy soy (10 to 15 grams of whole food soy) most days and tea (aim for at least 4 cups daily, 2 of them green tea).

9. Drink 1 cup organic carrot juice in the morning and 1 cup R.W. Knudsen Very Veggie Cocktail (low sodium) in the evening (or vice versa).

10. The number one preventable cause of cataracts and macular degeneration is smoking, so if you smoke, stop; avoid secondhand smoke as well.

11. Take Maxivision Whole Body Formula, or SFRx Daily Dose Packette plus 6 milligrams of supplemental lutein (such as Carlson Lutein, 6 mg; www.carlsonlabs.com), plus an EPA/DHA supplement (500 to 1000 milligrams a day for adult women and 1000 to 2000 milligrams a day for adult men).

16 Tips for Avoiding Alzheimer's Disease/Cognitive Decline

As we get older, we all have the kind of "senior moments" where we meet someone on the street we've known for twenty years—and greet him with a cheery, "Hey, there, buddy ..." because we cannot for the life of us remember his name.

These moments are not only embarrassing; they make us incredibly nervous and fearful that they are a sign of the kind of slippage we all fear the most—the kind from which there is no return. We've seen it in friends or relatives who begin by forgetting where they parked the car and end up in a world where they don't remember their own lives. It's a sad fact of some people's old age, but it doesn't have to be our destiny. There are many factors that contribute to mental decline and many steps you can take to help prevent it from happening, or at least to dramatically slow its progression. Here are sixteen of them:

1. Wear a helmet when riding a bicycle, motorcycle, skateboard, horse, and so on, as head trauma increases the risk for Alzheimer's disease.
2. Aim for a blood pressure reading of 115/80 or lower.
3. Aim for a fasting blood sugar level between 70 and 100 milligrams of glucose per deciliter of blood. See your health professional to get your blood sugar levels tested.
4. Aim for a total cholesterol level of less than 200 mg/dl and LDL-C of less than 100 mg/dl.
5. If you smoke, stop, and avoid exposure to second-hand smoke.
6. Keep your BMI and waist circumference within the normal range (see page 340 for BMI and waist circumference charts).
7. Have two to four servings (3 to 4 ounces or the size of a deck of cards) of wild Alaskan salmon or sidekicks per week. Your mother was right: Fish is

brain food. A number of studies have shown that omega-3s, especially from fish and fish oil, reduce the risk for dementia and cognitive decline. One important study followed eight hundred people ages sixty-five to ninety-four who initially did not have Alzheimer's disease. Researchers found that those who consumed fish at least once a week had a 60 percent reduced risk of developing Alzheimer's over the four years of the study as compared to participants who rarely or never ate fish.

8. Enjoy these other brain foods: blueberries or strawberries (1 to 2 cups a day); purple grape juice (4 to 8 ounces a day); spinach (2 cups raw or ½ cup to 1 cup cooked) or sidekicks five to seven days a week; and 1 ounce walnuts multiple times a week.

9. Include a high dietary intake of foods rich in vitamin C and E (see pages 257 and 258).

10. Include thirty to ninety minutes of physical activity five times a week.

11. Exercise your brain by reading, playing board games, playing musical instruments, dancing, socializing, and so on.

12. Get the lead out. In an environment where there are high amounts of lead and little iron in the diet, lead will be absorbed by young children, and even low levels of lead can cause a substantial reduction in IQ. Be sure your diet and especially your children's diets contain plenty of SuperFoods rich in iron and calcium. All iron is more bioavailable when you have vitamin C in the meal. Foods rich in iron include spinach, shiitake mushrooms, kidney beans, sesame seeds, pumpkin seeds, lentils, Swiss chard, tofu, green beans, kale, shrimp, broccoli, Brussels sprouts, soybeans, wheat germ, lima beans, green peas, skinless turkey breast, and lean red meat. Foods rich in calcium include collard greens, Swiss chard, kale, nonfat organic dairy products, low-fat cheese, fortified soymilk, broccoli, tofu, canned

sardines and wild salmon (with bones), green beans, green peas, and almonds.

13. Enjoy 1 serving of cruciferous veggies most days (½ cup raw or 1 cup cooked—½ to 1 baseball).

14. Include 500 to 1000 milligrams per day for adult females, 1000 to 2000 milligrams per day for adult males of fish oil supplement in your daily regimen.

15. Include 4 grams of whole grain bran a day (see the whole grain list on page 269).

16. Limit saturated fat intake by avoiding full-fat dairy and butter, and limit red meat intake to one serving (3 to 4 ounces or the size of a deck of cards) every seven to ten days.

Pay Yourself First

Not too long ago a stockbroker friend of mine gave me some advice: "We all have bills and obligations every month that have to be paid. But this should be your most important obligation: Pay yourself first. Put a little bit aside in a savings account. That's where your future lies." It's the same with SuperHealth. Every time you eat a blueberry or dine on wild salmon, every time you "green up" your life even in the smallest way, every time you get out of your house or from behind your desk and take a walk around the block, you're paying yourself first. You're building your life-savings account. And you are not the only beneficiary. Your children, your grandchildren, the world around you—everyone benefits. What could be better than that?

This book has been a tribute to my mom. But it's also a tribute to the mom in all of us—the part of us that knows instinctually in our hearts what's right, even if we may not want to deal with the reality. It's time to get back to the basics of good health that will bless us with longer, healthier lives. I congratulate you on taking this journey with me. I hope you picked up a few healthy tricks along the way, learned a thing or two, and, most of all, enjoyed yourself. Keep it up and don't give up.

This book has been all about making your life the best that it can be. Making it easy. Making it fun. The things I've asked you to do are simple things, small changes in the way you eat, the way you move, the way you look at the world. There's no excuse not to live the SuperHealth life. Whether you become an elite world-class "SuperHealther" or just a weekend warrior, picking up bits and pieces here and there, it will all do you good. Everybody can find a way to do this. Check out Dr. Steve's Daily Planner (page 229) for a quick snapshot of how I plan the foods I'm going to eat for the day to make sure I cover all the Super-Foods bases.

The goal from here is to make SuperHealth a habit. Once you've made something a habit, you don't have to think about it anymore. It's not just part of your life; it is your life. Make it fun. If it's not fun, you won't do it for a lifetime. This book is not about following a program for a few weeks to lose weight and feel energized; it's about a lifetime of good health. So here's to you, and here's to a super lifetime of better habits, better years, and SuperHealth! For the complete Week 6 Planner, see page 317.

◆ MEET SHIRLEY HARPER ◆

A Dancer at Heart

Shirley Harper has been a dancer all her life. "My mother used to say to me, 'Shirley, there's more to life than dancing. You'd better learn that.' But I never did," says Harper. "I'm eighty years old, and I still dance all the time—the Cha Cha, the Rumba. All of that. If I were younger, I bet I could keep up with *Dancing with the Stars*."

You can't argue with that. Shirley Harper is always on the go. She still plays golf and scores pretty well for her age, if she does say so herself. Give her a minute and she'll share with you her happy childhood memories of growing up in Williamsport, Pennsylvania, the home of the Little League World Championship. "There were no computers when I was growing up, none of that nonsense. We kids always went outside to play. I went roller skating and ice skating and tobogganing and did all kinds of other activities," she says. "Kids today don't get out and get exercise, and I think being active when you're young contributes to long life. We lived in a little vacuum back then. We didn't know all the things kids know today, but we had a very good life."

Even the difficult parts of life are not enough to keep Harper down. In 1980 she lost her husband and son in a plane crash. She didn't think she'd make it through this tragic time, but she managed with the help of friends and a "keep going" attitude. "I learned that you have to pull yourself together and get up and do things and live the rest of your life."

"I'm happy in my life," she says. "I exercise and I eat the proper food. I never go on a diet. I eat in moderation. I eat the things I want to eat, so I'm not unhappy. I have an occasional cocktail, but I don't get carried away. And I'm always on the go. I keep up with the news so I can converse with people, and I keep myself active. Who wants to sit at home and watch television—except for *Dancing with the Stars*, of course."

The SuperHealth Reference Guide

PART II.

The
SuperHealth
Reference
Guide

9

Dr. Steve's Daily Planner

People are always asking me what I eat on a daily basis, so I thought I'd share that information with you here. The 6-Step, 6-Week plan that is the basis of this book was designed to introduce you slowly to the SuperFoods and to their health relevance, and to build one week upon the next. Now that you understand the Super-Health philosophy, you can use this daily planner to make particular choices for the day, or mix and match from any of the six-step daily planners.

I'm not going to give you a list of what I have for breakfast, lunch, and dinner each day. Instead I'm going to tell you how I think about food: Every day I try to make sure that I have at least one SuperFood that protects one organ system or helps prevent one of the six major diseases. So I think, "What can I eat today that's good for my skin, or my eyes, or my brain, or my heart? What do I need in order to protect myself against cancer or inflammation or to help control my blood sugar?" I try to eat at least one food from each category every day to cover all my bases.

It's not that difficult to do. For one thing, many foods cover many bases. For instance, most foods that are good for the heart are good for the brain and eyes. So if you choose to eat wild salmon on any particular day, you've already covered these three categories. And selecting from the twenty-five SuperFoods and all their sidekicks gives you an incredible variety from which to choose. The best part is that your day will be so filled with healthy, satisfying SuperFoods that you won't be craving (or have room for) those sugary snacks and carb-filled meals you might otherwise consume.

As I have done throughout the book, I am including serving sizes and suggested frequencies for the foods listed here. When I suggest that you have a food daily (for instance, spinach or sidekicks), it means you should be aiming for that goal. But if you miss one day, there's no need to panic. You'll be just fine having green leafies five or six days a week instead of seven. You may also find that one food or group of foods is repeated in more than one category. That's because SuperFoods are good for so many different things.

And while you're planning your food for the day, don't forget the lifestyle choices that are part of the SuperHealth program. I try to get between sixty and ninety minutes of exercise a day, six days a week. I don't always do it all at once: There are plenty of exercises in the book that can be done anytime you have a few minutes to spare and/or while you're doing something else. My goal is to get myself moving as often as possible during the day, enjoying myself and burning calories at the same time. I try to get my seven hours of sleep every night so I can wake up fresh and refreshed and ready for another SuperHealth day.

Skin Health:

Tip of the day: Try my "natural sunscreen/tanner"—1 cup of organic carrot juice with breakfast and one cup of R.W. Knudsen Very Veggie Vegetable Cocktail (low sodium) with dinner (or vice versa).

SuperFood/ Nutrient	Amount	Sidekicks	Comments
Pumpkin	1 cup (1 baseball)	Carrots, butternut squash	Have raw or cooked carrots, or

SuperFood/ Nutrient	Amount	Sidekicks	Comments
			any recipe with pumpkin (such as Marlaina's Pumpkin Pie Smoothie, page 286) or butternut squash.
Tomatoes	1 serving of processed tomatoes, such as 1 to 2 tablespoons of tomato paste or sidekicks a day and multiple servings of fresh tomatoes	Watermelon, pink grapefruit, Japanese persimmons, red-fleshed papayas, strawberry guavas	Very Veggie Cocktail is tomato juice–based, so you can substitute other sources of cooked tomatoes, such as tomato paste, marinara sauce, ketchup, canned tomatoes, and taco sauce.
Dark chocolate	About 100 calories most days		Adjust your calorie intake and exercise appropriately. Try Dr. Steve's Hot Chocolate recipe, page 280.

Eye Health:

Tip of the day: Spinach is the most important SuperFood for the eyes, so I try to have a SuperHealth Spinach Salad (page 280) almost every day. It's good for every body system, not just your eyes, so it's a no-brainer for me.

SuperFood/ Nutrient	Amount	Sidekicks	Comments
Lutein	1 cup steamed (1 baseball) or	Spinach, kale, collard greens,	Green leafy vegetables are a

(continued)

SuperFood/ Nutrient	Amount	Sidekicks	Comments
Lutein (*cont.*)	2 cups raw, five to seven days a week	Swiss chard, arugula, mustard greens, turnip greens, bok choy, romaine lettuce, seaweed, purslane	great source of lutein, important for eye health.
Zeaxanthin	1 cup (1 baseball), five to seven days a week	Orange bell pepper, goji berries (¼ cup), yellow corn, cornmeal (¼ cup)	Whole Foods 365 Organic Yellow Corn Tortilla Chips and Corn Strips are good low-sodium choices. Both lutein and zeaxanthin are good for skin health as well.

Heart Health:

Tip of the day: Omega-3 fatty acids, found in wild salmon and its sidekicks, are essential for heart health. I take an omega-3 supplement (see page 261) almost every day—but especially on the days I'm not having fish.

SuperFood/ Nutrient	Amount	Sidekicks	Comments
Wild salmon	3 to 4 ounces (deck of cards), two to four times a week	Alaskan/northern halibut, canned chunk light or albacore tuna, mackerel, sardines, farmed trout, herring, oysters and clams (farmed or wild)	If you're looking for a delicious way to eat salmon, try the recipe for Moosh-a-Magulla on page 282.

SuperFood/ Nutrient	Amount	Sidekicks	Comments
Whole grains	10 grams of whole grain fiber a day	Oats, oat bran, wheat germ, ground flaxseed, barley, rye, amaranth, corn bran, wheat, millet, quinoa, triticale, wild rice, kamut, spelt, brown rice, buckwheat, bulgar wheat, yellow corn	Women need about 32 grams of dietary fiber a day and men need about 45; 10 of those grams should come from whole grains, and ideally 4 of those should come from whole grain bran (oat bran, wheat bran, corn bran).
Blueberries	1 to 2 cups daily (1 to 2 baseballs)	Purple grapes, cranberries, boysenberries, raspberries, strawberries, fresh currants, blackberries, cherries, goji berries, açai berries, lingonberries, and all other varieties of fresh, frozen, or freeze-dried berries	Bathe your meals in berries and/or sidekicks. I try to have berries in one form or another at almost every meal. This will help raise your good cholesterol (HDLC), lower inflammatory markers (CRP), and will thin your blood just like aspirin.

Brain Health:

Tip of the day: Two of the best food categories for the brain are the ones high in vitamin E and vitamin C.

SuperFood/ Nutrient	Amount	Sidekicks	Comments
Walnuts	1 layer on your palm, five days a week	Almonds, pistachios, sesame seeds, peanuts, pumpkin and sunflower seeds, macadamia nuts, pecans, hazelnuts, cashews	Walnuts in the shell are good for portion control. It takes so long to get at each nut that it seems like you're eating more than you really are.
Oranges	1 medium orange (1 baseball) daily	Lemons, white and pink grapefruits, kumquats, tangerines, limes	Like the taste of orange? Try the recipe for Orange-Poppyseed Dressing on page 281.
Kiwis	1 kiwi, multiple times a week	Brazilian pineapple, or strawberry guava	If you want maximum nutrition from your kiwi, don't skip the skin. Beneath that fuzz lies a treasure trove of nutrients and fiber, so rinse it off and bite right in!

Skeletal Strength:

Tip of the day: While yogurt supplies much of the calcium you need for bone health, you also need potassium and vitamin K to keep those bones strong and healthy.

SuperFood/ Nutrient	Amount	Sidekicks	Comments
Yogurt (nonfat)	1 to 2 cups (1 to 2 baseballs) most days	Kefir, soy yogurt	I often buy "fruit-on-the-bottom" yogurt and don't eat the bottom—that way I get the taste of the fruit without the sugar.
Potassium	Aim for 8000 milligrams daily	See the list of potassium all-stars, page 275.	Follow the SuperHealth food planners and you'll reach your potassium goal in no time.
Vitamin K	1 serving (1 cup steamed [1 baseball] or 2 cups raw five to seven days a week) of green leafies more than meets the requirement	Spinach, kale, collard greens, broccoli, Swiss chard, arugula, mustard greens, turnip greens, bok choy, romaine lettuce, orange bell peppers, carrots, string beans, asparagus	Kale, collards greens, spinach, and turnip greens have the highest amounts of vitamin K.
Skinless turkey breast	3 to 4 ounces (1 deck of cards), three to four times a week	Skinless chicken breast	Check out the terrific turkey recipes on pages 283–84.

Anticancer Foods:

Tip of the day: The foods under the broccoli heading may look very familiar—they're all rich in vitamin K.

SuperFood/ Nutrient	Amount	Sidekicks	Comments
Broccoli	1 cup steamed (1 baseball) or 2 cups raw five to seven days a week	Spinach, kale, collard greens, Swiss chard, arugula, mustard greens, turnip greens, bok choy, romaine lettuce, red and green cabbage, cauliflower, rutabaga, kohlrabi, broccoflower, arugula, watercress	I want to be sure to include cruciferous veggies every day so I know I'm getting an anticancer powerhouse.
Onions	⅛ to ¼ medium onion or sidekick most days	Scallions, shallots, leeks, chives, garlic	I eat onions (or sidekicks) almost every day—sometimes raw in a salad or sliced on a sandwich, sometimes cooked in a sauce or vegetable stir-fry.
Garlic	To taste, as often as you like, at least cooked.	Scallions, shallots, leeks, chives, onions	Here's a hint about cooking with garlic: It mellows the longer it is cooked. Adding garlic at the end of cooking will give a stronger taste than when added earlier.

Anti-inflammatory Foods:

Tip of the day: Salmon and berries make repeat visits here because we just can't get enough of those omega-3s and polyphenols!

SuperFood/ Nutrient	Amount	Sidekicks	Comments
Wild salmon	3 to 4 ounces (1 deck of cards), two to four times a week	Alaskan/northern halibut, canned chunk light or albacore tuna, mackerel, sardines, farmed trout, herring, oysters and clams (farmed or wild)	Add some canned tuna or Alaskan salmon to the SuperHealth Spinach Salad (page 280) and you've got a great lunch or dinner.
Blueberries	1 to 2 cups daily (1 to 2 baseballs)	Purple grapes, cranberries, boysenberries, raspberries, strawberries, fresh currants, blackberries, cherries, goji berries, açai berries, lingonberries, and all other varieties of fresh, frozen, or freeze-dried berries	Remember that you can drink 100% berry juices (one to two ½-cup servings) instead of fresh or frozen whole fruits.
Pomegranate	½ cup to 1 cup (4 to 8 ounces) 100% pomegranate juice, five to seven times a week	Plums (fresh or dried)	100% pomegranate juice can be too strong for some tastes; you may like berry combos instead (such as pom-cherry, pom-blueberry, pom-cranberry)

(continued)

SuperFood/ Nutrient	Amount	Sidekicks	Comments
Extra virgin olive oil	1 to 2 tablespoons most days	Canola oil	For a flavorful orange-poppyseed salad dressing using EVOO, see page 281.
Spices	As much as you like, to taste, as often as you like	Anise, black pepper, caraway seeds, cayenne pepper, cumin, fennel, ginger, fenugreek, licorice, marjoram, nutmeg, oregano, rosemary, saffron, sage, thyme, turmeric	. . . and any other spices you don't see on this list.

Foods for Controlling Blood Sugar:

Tip of the day: We now know that controlling your blood sugar may be the key to living a longer and healthier life, so I'm conscientious about including a variety of beans and whole grains in my diet.

SuperFood/ Nutrient	Amount	Sidekicks	Comments
Beans	At least four ½-cup (½ baseball) servings a week	All beans, including pinto, kidney, navy, great Northern, lima, and garbanzo, lentils, string beans (or any green beans), sugar snap peas, green peas	Beans are a good choice if you're trying to lose weight because they provide bulk without adding a lot of calories. They fill you up, minimizing hunger and maintaining high energy levels throughout the day.

SuperFood/ Nutrient	Amount	Sidekicks	Comments
Whole grains	10 grams of whole grain fiber a day	Oats, oat bran, wheat germ, ground flaxseed, barley, rye, amaranth, corn bran, wheat, millet, quinoa, triticale, wild rice, kamut, spelt, brown rice, buckwheat, bulgar wheat, yellow corn	Here they are again. The fact that they show up so often gives you an idea of just how essential they are to the SuperHealth program. They also decrease our risk for multiple inflammatory diseases.
Apples	Try to eat an apple (or pear) a day (1 medium—size of a baseball)	Pears	An apple a day helps keep diabetes away. Apples are full of healthy polyphenols, fiber, potassium, and vitamin C.
Honey	1 to 2 teaspoons multiple times a week		Remember that the flavonoids in honey help our bodies regulate blood sugar—and the darker the honey, the more flavonoids it contains.

Nutrient Boosters:

Tip of the day: If you want to give your body a little help in absorbing all the nutrients included in SuperFoods, you need to include the healthy fats in the chart below. Black pepper also helps increase the body's ability to absorb the bioactive "goodies" in SuperFoods.

SuperFood/ Nutrient	Amount	Sidekicks	Comments
Avocados	⅓ to ½ avocado multiple times a week	Asparagus, artichokes	If you're watching your weight, be sure to adjust your calorie count for the day when you add avocado to your diet, as it is a healthy but calorie-dense food.
Extra virgin olive oil	1 to 2 tablespoons most days	Canola oil	Look for first-cold-pressed EVOO, which is a higher quality of olive oil that is naturally lower in acidity.
Nuts and seeds	1 layer on your palm, five days a week	Walnuts, almonds, pistachios, sesame seeds, peanuts, pumpkin and sunflower seeds, macadamia nuts, pecans, hazelnuts, cashews	Remember to keep unshelled nuts in the fridge so they stay fresh longer.
Wild salmon	3 to 4 ounces (1 deck of cards), two to four times a week	Alaskan/northern halibut, canned chunk light or albacore tuna, mackerel, sardines, farmed trout, herring,	If you're looking for an excellent source of frozen fish, try www.vitalchoice .com or Whole

SuperFood/ Nutrient	Amount	Sidekicks	Comments
		oysters and clams (farmed or wild)	Foods Market.
Black pepper	To taste, as often as you like		Black pepper enhances digestion, reduces gas, stimulates the breakdown of fat cells, increases absorption of various beneficial nutrients and phytonutrients, and exerts substantial antioxidant, anti-inflammatory, and antimicrobial effects.

Daily Supplements:

Tip of the day: It would be ideal if we got all the nutrients we needed from food every day. However, living in the real modern world doesn't always allow for that. In order to protect my body in as many ways as possible, I take the supplements below almost every day.

SuperFood/ Nutrient	Amount	Sidekicks	Comments
Multivitamin	Follow label instructions		My favorite choices are MaxiVision Whole Body Formula or Daily Dose Packettes (www.superfoodsrx .com).

(continued)

SuperFood/ Nutrient	Amount	Sidekicks	Comments
EPA/DHA	500 to 1000 mgs a day for adult women and 1000 to 2000 mg for adult men		I take EPA/DHA several times a day, especially on the days I am not having a fish meal.
Vitamin D	600 to 2000 IU of D_3 daily		Be sure to also include foods rich in vitamin D in your daily diet. For foods rich in vitamin D, see page 256.

Daily Beverages:

Tip of the day: Drink up! We all need plenty of liquid every day. I mix and match from the list below.

SuperFood/ Nutrient	Amount	Sidekicks	Comments
Tea	4 cups daily	White, green, black, oolong, rooibos	These days there are hundreds of varieties of tea available at your local supermarket and online. Try different flavors, find the ones you like, and keep drinking. And don't forget, there's nothing more refreshing

SuperFood/ Nutrient	Amount	Sidekicks	Comments
			than a glass of iced tea on a hot day. Add a bit of citrus to boost the bioavailability of tea's phyto-nutrients.
Hot chocolate	1 cup several times a week		See my recipe on page 280.
100% fruit juices	½ cup (4 ounces) twice daily	Whole fruits	My five favorites are pomegranate, Concord grape, blueberry, cranberry, and cherry.
Water	At least five 8-ounce glasses daily		Bottled or tap, be sure you keep yourself hydrated throughout the day.

10

The 25 SuperFoods and 15 SuperNutrients

Apples

A source of:

- Polyphenols
- Fiber
- Vitamin C
- Potassium

Sidekick: Pears
Try to eat: 1 apple a day (1 baseball)

Avocados

A source of:

- Monounsaturated fatty acids
- Fiber
- Magnesium
- Folate
- Vitamin E
- Carotenoids
- Glutathione
- Beta-sitosterol

- Chlorophyll
- Polyphenols
- Lutein

Sidekicks: Asparagus, artichokes, extra virgin olive oil

Try to eat: ⅓ to ½ of an avocado multiple times a week

Beans

A source of:

- Low-fat protein
- Fiber
- B vitamins
- Iron
- Folate
- Potassium
- Magnesium
- Phytonutrients

Sidekicks: All beans are included in this SuperFood category—some examples include pinto, kidney, navy, great Northern, lima, and garbanzo beans (chickpeas), lentils, string beans (or green beans), sugar snap peas, green peas

Try to eat: At least four ½ cup (½ baseball) servings a week

Blueberries

A source of:

- Synergy of multiple nutrients and phytonutrients
- Polyphenols (proanthocyanins, anthocyanins, quercetin, catechins)
- Salicylic acid
- Carotenoids
- Fiber

- Folate
- Vitamin C
- Vitamin E
- Potassium
- Manganese
- Magnesium
- Iron
- Resveratrol
- Riboflavin
- Niacin
- Phytoestrogens
- Low calories

Sidekicks: purple grapes, cranberries, boysenberries, raspberries, strawberries, fresh currants, blackberries, cherries, and all other varieties of fresh, frozen, or freeze-dried berries

Try to eat: 1 to 2 cups (1 to 2 baseballs) a day

Broccoli

A source of:

- Sulforaphane
- Indoles
- Folate
- Fiber
- Calcium
- Vitamin C
- Beta-carotene
- Lutein/zeaxanthin
- Vitamin K

Sidekicks: Brussels sprouts, red and green cabbage, kale, turnips, cauliflower, collard greens, bok choy, mustard greens, Swiss chard, rutabaga, kohlrabi, broccoflower, arugula, watercress, daikon, wasabi, liverwort

Try to eat: ½ cup to 1 cup (½ to 1 baseball) most days

Chocolate (Dark)

A source of:

- Fiber
- Magnesium
- Polyphenols

Try to eat: About 100 calories dark chocolate a day, adjusting your calorie intake and exercise appropriately

Cinnamon

Try to eat: As much as you like, to taste, as often as you like

Dried Fruits

Raisins, prunes, dates, dried figs, blueberries, cranberries, cherries, currants, apricots, and apples (all no sugar added).

A source of:

- Fiber
- Phytonutrients
- Potassium

Try to eat: 2 heaping tablespoons (1 shot glass) three to four times a week or follow the package label for serving size

Extra Virgin Olive Oil (EVOO)

A source of:

- Monounsaturated fatty acids
- Vitamin E
- Carotenoids
- Polyphenols
- Phytosterols

Sidekick: Canola oil
Try to eat: 1 to 2 tablespoons (½ to 1 shot glass) most days

Garlic

A source of:

- Organosulfur compounds (75 total, with allicin the most active)
- Saponins
- Polyphenols
- Selenium
- Arginine
- Vitamin C
- Potassium

Sidekicks: scallions, shallots, leeks, onions
Try to eat: To taste, multiple times a week

Honey

A source of 181 different substances, including:

- Polyphenols
- Salicylates
- Oligosaccharides

Try to eat: 1 to 2 teaspoons multiple times a week

Kiwis

A source of:

- Vitamin C
- Folate
- Vitamin E
- Potassium
- Fiber
- Carotenoids (primarily lutein and zeaxanthin)

- Polyphenols
- Chlorophyll
- Glutathione
- Pectin
- Low glycemic index

Sidekicks: Brazilian pineapple, or strawberry guava
Try to eat: Multiple times a week

Oats

A source of:

- Fiber
- Beta glucan
- Low calories
- Protein
- Magnesium
- Potassium
- Zinc
- Copper
- Manganese
- Selenium
- Thiamin

SuperSidekicks: wheat germ, ground flaxseed
Sidekicks: brown rice, barley, wheat, buckwheat, rye, millet, bulgar wheat, amaranth, quinoa, triticale, kamut, yellow corn, wild rice, spelt, couscous
Try to eat: Whole grain foods that contain a daily minimum of 10 grams of whole grain fiber

Onions

A source of:

- Selenium
- Fructans (including inulin)
- Vitamin E
- Vitamin C

- Potassium
- Diallyl sulfide
- Saponins
- Fiber
- Polyphenols

Sidekicks: garlic, scallions, shallots, leeks, chives
Try to eat: ⅛ to ¼ medium onion or sidekick most days

Oranges

A source of:

- Vitamin C
- Fiber
- Folate
- Limonene
- Potassium
- Polyphenols
- Pectin

Sidekicks: lemons, white and pink grapefruits, kumquats, tangerines, limes
Try to eat: 1 serving a day

Pomegranates

A source of:

- Viamin B$_6$
- Vitamin C
- Polyphenols
- Potassium

Sidekicks: plums (fresh or dried)
Try to eat: ½ cup to 1 cup (4 to 8 ounces) of 100% pomegranate juice multiple times a week

Pumpkin

A source of:

- Alpha-carotene
- Beta-carotene
- High fiber
- Low calories
- Vitamins C and E
- Potassium
- Magnesium
- Pantothenic acid

Sidekicks: carrots, butternut squash, sweet potatoes, orange bell peppers

Try to eat: ½ cup (½ baseball) five to seven days a week

Salmon (Wild)

A source of:

- Marine-derived omega-3 fatty acids
- B vitamins
- Calcium (when canned with bones)
- Selenium
- Vitamin D
- Potassium
- Protein
- Carotenoids

Sidekicks: Alaskan/northern halibut, canned chunk light or albacore tuna, mackerel, sardines, herring, farmed trout, oysters, and clams (farmed or wild)

Try to eat: 3 to 4 ounces (1 deck of cards) two to four times a week

Soy

A source of:

- Phytoestrogens
- Plant-derived omega-3 fatty acids
- Vitamin E
- B vitamins (thiamin, riboflavin, B_6)
- Iron
- Potassium
- Folate
- Magnesium
- Selenium
- Saponins
- Phytates
- Phytosterols
- Lunasin
- Excellent nonmeat protein alternative

Sidekicks (forms of soy): tofu, soymilk, soy yogurt, soy nuts, edamame, tempeh, miso

Try to eat: Aim for 10 to 15 grams of soy protein a day (this equals 30 to 50 milligrams of isoflavones a day; isoflavones from the whole food sources listed above)

Spinach

A source of:

- Synergy of multiple nutrients/phytonutrients
- Low calories
- Lutein/zeaxanthin
- Beta-carotene
- Plant-derived omega-3 fatty acids
- Glutathione
- Alpha-lipoic acid
- Vitamins C and E
- B vitamins (thiamin, riboflavin, B_6, folate)
- Minerals: calcium, iron, magnesium, manganese, and zinc

- Polyphenols
- Betaine
- Coenzyme Q_{10}

Sidekicks: kale, collard greens, Swiss chard, arugula, mustard greens, turnip greens, bok choy, romaine lettuce, orange bell peppers, seaweed

Try to eat: 1 cup steamed (1 baseball) or 2 cups raw (2 baseballs) most days

Tea

A source of:

- Flavonoids
- Fluoride
- No calories

Try to drink: 1 to 4 cups a day or more

Tomatoes

A source of:

- Lycopene
- Low calories
- Vitamin C
- Alpha-carotene and beta-carotene
- Phytuene and phytofluence
- Potassium
- B vitamins (B_6, niacin, folate, thiamin, pantothenic acid)
- Chromium
- Biotin
- Fiber

Sidekicks: watermelon, pink grapefruit, Japanese persimmons, red-fleshed papayas, strawberry guava

Try to eat: 1 serving of cooked or processed tomatoes

or sidekicks a day and multiple servings a week of fresh tomatoes

Turkey (Skinless Breast)

A source of:

- Low-fat protein
- Riboflavin
- Niacin
- Vitamin B_6
- Vitamin B_{12}
- Iron
- Selenium
- Zinc

Sidekicks: skinless chicken breast
Try to eat: 3 to 4 ounces (1 deck of cards) three to four times a week

Walnuts

A source of:

- Plant-derived omega-3 fatty acids
- Vitamin E
- Magnesium
- Polyphenols
- Protein
- Fiber
- Potassium
- Plant sterols
- Vitamin B_6
- Arginine
- Resveratrol
- Melatonin

Sidekicks: almonds, pistachios, sesame seeds, peanuts, pumpkin and sunflower seeds, macadamia nuts, pecans, hazelnuts, cashews

Try to eat: 1 ounce (1 layer on your palm) five times a week

Yogurt (Preferably Nonfat and Organic)

A source of:

- Live active cultures
- Complete protein
- Calcium
- Vitamin B$_2$ (riboflavin)
- Vitamin B$_{12}$
- Potassium
- Magnesium
- Zinc
- Conjugated linolenic acid

Sidekicks: kefir, soy yogurt, DanActive Immunity, Sustenex capsules

Try to eat: 1 to 2 cups (1 to 2 baseballs) most days

THE 15 SUPERNUTRIENTS

If you analyze all the most health-promoting, disease-preventing, anti-aging, risk-factor-limiting diets in the world, fifteen nutrients consistently turn up. These nutrients are associated with reducing a wide range of chronic ailments. Countless studies demonstrate that the higher your level of these nutrients, the slower you age and the less chance you have of suffering from chronic disease. Here is a list of these SuperNutrients, along with the richest food sources of the "super fifteen."

If you have a bleeding or clotting problem, or if you are taking anticoagulants, consult your health-care professional before adopting any of the recommendations listed here.

Vitamin D: The SuperLongevity Nutrient

The news about vitamin D is so good that it's almost too good to be true. If you get enough, it helps combat almost every major form of disease (heart disease, cancer, you name it!).

Aim for consuming two foods containing vitamin D_2 or D_3 daily (all nonfortified vitamin D found in foods is vitamin D_3). There is no recommended daily amount of vitamin D from food, so be sure to expose skin (you choose which parts) to sunlight for fifteen minutes at least three times a week, remembering that there is no vitamin D production from sunlight during the winter months in many parts of the world, and take a vitamin D_3 supplement daily, with teens and older aiming for 600 to 2000 IU of supplemental D_3 daily.

- 1 tablespoon cod liver oil = 1360 IU
- 3.5 ounces wild sockeye salmon (Alaskan) = 670 IU
- 3.5 ounces albacore tuna = 540 IU
- 3.5 ounces wild silver salmon (Alaskan) = 425 IU
- 3 ounces canned pink salmon = 360 IU
- 3 ounces canned sardines = 250 IU
- 3 ounces canned mackerel = 244 IU
- 3.5 ounces wild king salmon (Alaskan) = 222 IU
- 3 ounces canned white tuna = 200 IU
- 4 ounces shrimp = 162 IU
- 1 cup milk (fortified) = 100 IU
- 1 cup soymilk (fortified) = 100 IU
- 1 cup orange juice (fortified) = 100 IU
- 4 ounces cod = 64 IU
- 1 cup cereal (fortified) = 40 IU
- 1 egg yolk = 20 IU

Vitamin C

Aim for at least 350 milligrams a day from a combination of the following foods:

- 1 large yellow bell pepper = 341 mg
- 1 large red bell pepper = 312 mg
- 1 guava = 165 mg
- 1 large green bell pepper = 132 mg
- 1 cup fresh orange juice = 124 mg (97 mg a cup from frozen concentrate)
- 1 cup fresh sliced strawberries = 97 mg
- 1 cup fresh chopped broccoli = 79 mg
- 1 medium kiwi = 57 mg

Folic Acid

Aim for 400 micrograms a day from a combination of the following foods (in food folic acid is called folate):

- 1 cup cooked spinach = 263 mcg
- 1 cup cooked kidney beans = 230 mcg
- 1 cup boiled green soybeans = 200 mcg
- ½ cup soy nuts = 177 mcg
- 1 cup orange juice from frozen concentrate = 110 mcg
- 1 cup frozen chopped cooked broccoli = 103 mcg
- 4 cooked asparagus spears = 89 mcg

Selenium

Aim for 70 to 100 micrograms a day from a combination of the following foods:

- 3 ounces cooked Pacific oysters = 131 mcg
- 1 cup whole wheat flour = 85 mcg
- ½ can Pacific sardines = 75 mcg
- 1 dried Brazil nut = 68 to 91 mcg
- 3 ounces canned white tuna = 56 mcg
- 3 ounces cooked clams = 54 mcg

- 6 farmed oysters = 54 mcg
- 3 ounces roasted skinless turkey breast = 27 mcg

Vitamin E

Aim for at least 16 milligrams a day from a combination of the following foods:

- 2 tablespoons wheat germ oil = 41 mg
- 2 tablespoons canola oil = 13.6 mg
- 2 tablespoons peanut oil = 9.2 mg
- 1 ounce raw almonds (23 or 24) = 7.7 mg
- ¼ cup hulled dry-roasted sunflower seeds = 6.8 mg
- 2 tablespoons raw (untoasted) wheat germ = 5 mg
- 1 medium orange bell pepper = 4.3 mg
- 1 ounce hazelnuts (20 to 21) = 4.3 mg
- 2 tablespoons extra virgin olive oil = 4 mg
- 2 tablespoons peanut butter = 3.2 mg
- 1 cup blueberries = 2.8 mg
- 2 tablespoons soybean oil = 2.6 mg

Lycopene

Aim for 22 milligrams a day of this carotenoid from a combination of the following foods:

- 1 cup tomato sauce (canned) = 37 mg
- 1 cup R.W. Knudsen Very Veggie Low Sodium Vegetable Cocktail from concentrate = 22 mg
- 1 cup tomato juice = 22 mg
- 1 watermelon wedge = 13 mg
- 1 cup canned stewed tomatoes = 10.3 mg
- 1 tablespoon tomato paste = 4.6 mg
- 1 tablespoon ketchup = 2.9 mg
- ½ pink grapefruit = 1.8 mg

Keep in mind that lycopene is far more bioavailable from cooked or processed tomato products than raw.

The lycopene found in watermelon is very bioavailable. (To date we are not aware of any studies evaluating the absorption characteristics of other fruit sources of lycopene; presumably they are similar to watermelon.)

Lutein/Zeaxanthin

Aim for 12 milligrams a day of this carotenoid from a combination of the following foods:

LUTEIN SOURCES
- 1 cup cooked kale (chopped) = 23.7 mg
- 1 cup cooked spinach = 20.4 mg
- 1 cup cooked collard greens (chopped) = 14.6 mg
- 1 cup cooked turnip greens = 12.1 mg
- 1 cup cooked green peas = 4.2 mg
- 1 cup cooked broccoli (chopped) = 2.4 mg

ZEAXANTHIN SOURCES
- 1 medium orange bell pepper = 6.4 mg
- 25 to 35 dried goji berries = 1.45 mg
- 1 cup canned yellow corn = .9 mg
- 1 Japanese persimmon = .8 mg
- 1 cup degermed yellow cornmeal = .7 mg

Alpha-Carotene

Aim for 2.4 milligrams a day of this carotenoid from a combination of the following foods:

- 1 cup canned pumpkin = 11.7 mg
- 1 cup cooked carrots (sliced) = 6.6 mg
- 10 raw baby carrots = 3.8 mg
- 1 cup cooked butternut squash (cubed) = 2.3 mg
- 1 large orange bell pepper = .3 mg
- 1 cup cooked collard greens (chopped) = .2 mg

Beta-Carotene

Aim for 6 milligrams a day of this carotenoid from a combination of the following foods:

- 1 cup canned pumpkin = 17 mg
- 1 cup cooked cooked carrots (sliced) = 13 mg
- 1 cup cooked spinach = 11.3 mg
- 1 cup cooked chopped kale = 10.6 mg
- 1 cup cooked butternut squash (cubed) = 9.4 mg
- 1 cup cooked collard greens (chopped) = 9.2 mg

Beta-Cryptoxanthin

Aim for at least 1 milligram a day of this carotenoid from a combination of the following foods:

- 1 cup cooked butternut squash (cubed) = 6.4 mg
- 1 cup cooked red bell pepper (strips) = 2.8 mg
- 1 Japanese persimmon (2.5 inches in diameter) = 2.4 mg
- 1 cup mashed papaya = 1.8 mg
- 1 large red bell pepper (raw) = .8 mg
- 1 cup fresh tangerine juice = .5 mg
- 1 medium tangerine = .3 mg

Glutathione

Optimum daily recommendation amounts are not yet known. Foods high in glutathione include:

- Asparagus
- Watermelon
- Avocados
- Walnuts
- Grapefruits
- Peanut butter
- Oatmeal
- Broccoli
- Oranges
- Spinach

Resveratrol

Optimum daily recommendation amounts are not yet known. Data suggests that this phytonutrient plays a role in preventing inflammation and cancer and most likely has cardio-protective activity. Foods high in resveratrol include:

- Blueberries
- Peanuts (especially the skin)
- Purple grape skins
- Red wine
- Purple grape juice
- Cranberries/cranberry juice

Fiber

Optimum daily amounts are 32 grams of fiber a day for women and 45 grams of fiber a day for men. Foods high in fiber include:

- 1 cup cooked black beans = 15 g
- ¼ cup dried pinto beans = 14 g
- 1 cup cooked garbanzo beans = 13 g
- ¼ cup dried lentils = 9 g
- 1 cup fresh raspberries = 8 g

(Also consult the SuperHealth High-Fiber Choices list on page 264.)

Omega-3 Fatty Acids

The Food and Nutrition Board of the Institute of Medicine, the National Academies, recently set an adequate intake of 1.6 grams per day of plant-derived omega-3s (alpha-linolenic acid, ALA) for adult men and 1.1 grams per day for adult women. They set a target amount of marine-derived omega-3s (EPA/DHA) of 160 milligrams per day for adult men and 110 milligrams per day for adult women.

I agree with the Food and Nutrition Board's daily ALA recommendations (they are great minimums; if you reach higher daily intake levels eating the Super-Health way, that is okay). My personal recommendations for marine-derived omega-3s are 500 to 1000 milligrams per day for adult women and 1000 to 2000 milligrams per day for adult men.

EPA/DHA = Primarily marine-derived omega-3 food sources

- 3 ounces cooked Chinook (king) salmon = 1.5 g
- 3 ounces sockeye salmon = 1 g
- 3 ounces farmed rainbow trout = 1 g
- 1 can sardines = .9 g
- 3 ounces canned white tuna in water = .7 g

Other foods: SuperFoodsRx Premium Dark Chocolate and SuperFoodsRx Pizza are additional sources of EPA/DHA.

Alpha-linolenic acid (ALA) = Plant-derived omega-3 food sources

OILS
- 1 tablespoon canola oil = 1.3 g
- 1 tablespoon walnut oil = 1.4 g
- 1 tablespoon soybean oil = .7 g

OTHER FOODS
- 1 cup cooked spinach = .2 g
- 1 cup cooked collard greens = .2 g
- 1 ounce (14 halves) walnuts = 2.6 g
- 1 tablespoon flaxseed = 2.2 g
- ½ cup dry-roasted soy nuts = 1.2 g
- ½ cup wheat germ = .5 g
- 1 omega-3 egg = .15 to .25 g; check the carton

Polyphenols

Optimum daily recommended amounts for this class of phytonutrients have not yet been determined. The following foods and beverages have significant amounts of polyphenols:

WHOLE FOODS
- Berries
- Dates, figs
- Prunes
- Kale, spinach
- Parsley, dried parsley
- Apples with skin
- Citrus
- Grapes
- Whole grains
- Nuts and seeds
- Legumes

JAMS
The highest polyphenol content of the jams we tested:

- Trader Joe's Organic Blueberry Fruit Spread
- Knott's Berry Farm Pure Boysenberry Preserves
- Trader Joe's Organic Blackberry Fruit Spread

BEVERAGES
- Green, black, white, rooibos, or oolong tea
- Soymilk
- 100% fruit juices (berry, pomegranate, Concord grape, cherry, apple, citrus, prune)

The highest polyphenol content of the 100% fruit juices we tested:

- Odwalla C Monster
- Trader Joe's 100% Unfiltered Concord Grape Juice
- R.W. Knudsen 100% Just Pomegranate Juice

11

All-Stars: High-Fiber and Low-Sodium Food Choices, Plus Sources of Betaine, Choline, and Potassium

SUPERHEALTH HIGH-FIBER CHOICES

Bread
- Bran for Life Bread: 5 grams fiber per slice, 80 calories
- Food for Life Ezekiel 4:9 Sprouted Grain Bread: 3 grams fiber per slice, 80 calories
- Healthseed Spelt with pumpkin, flax, sesame and sunflower seeds (Wheat Free, Yeast Free): 5 grams fiber per slice, 88 calories
- Julian Bakery Cinnamon Almond Raisin Bread: 12 grams fiber per slice, 137 calories
- Julian Bakery Manna from Heaven: 9 grams fiber per slice, 110 calories

Cereals
- Barbara's Grain Shop High Fiber Cereal Medley: 8 grams fiber per ⅔ cup, 90 calories
- Bob's Red Mill Oat Bran Hot Cereal: 5 grams fiber per ⅓ cup, 120 calories
- Bob's Red Mill Wheat Bran: 6 grams fiber per ¼ cup, 30 calories

- Bob's Red Mill Whole Ground Flaxseed Meal: 4 grams fiber per 2 tablespoons, 60 calories
- General Mills Fiber One Bran Cereal: 14 grams fiber per ½ cup, 60 calories
- Kashi Go Lean High Protein, High Fiber Cereal: 10 grams fiber per ¾ cup, 140 calories
- Kellogg's All-Bran Buds: 13 grams fiber per ½ cup, 70 calories
- Kellogg's All-Bran (Extra Fiber): 13 grams fiber per ½ cup, 70 calories
- Kellogg's All-Bran Flakes: 10 grams fiber per ½ cup, 80 calories
- Kellogg's Complete Wheat Bran Flakes: 5 grams fiber per ¾ cup, 90 calories
- Mother's Toasted Wheat Germ: 2 grams fiber per 2 tablespoons, 50 calories
- Nature's Path Flax Plus Multibran Cereal: 7 grams fiber per ¾ cup, 100 calories
- Nature's Path Flax Plus Raisin Bran: 11 grams fiber per ¾ cup, 180 calories
- Nature's Path Heritage Muesli with Raspberries and Hazelnuts: 6 grams fiber per ½ cup, 220 calories
- Nature's Path Optimum Zen Cereal—Cranberry Ginger: 10 grams fiber per ¾ cup, 200 calories
- Post 100% Bran: 9 grams fiber per ⅓ cup, 80 calories
- Post Shredded Wheat: 6 grams fiber per 2 biscuits, 160 calories
- Post Shredded Wheat 'N Bran: 8 grams fiber per ½ cup, 200 calories
- Quaker Oat Bran Hot Cereal: 6 grams fiber per ½ cup, 150 calories
- Simply Fiber: 14 grams fiber per 1 cup, 100 calories
- Uncle Sam Cereal (Whole-Grain Wheat and Flaxseed): 10 grams fiber per 1 cup, 190 calories

Crackers and Crispbread

- Ak-Mak 100% Stone Ground Whole Wheat Sesame Crackers: 3.5 grams per 5 crackers, 116 calories
- Health Valley Amaranth Graham Crackers: 3 grams fiber per 6 crackers, 120 calories

- Health Valley Oat Bran Graham Crackers: 3 grams fiber per 6 crackers, 120 calories
- Health Valley Rice Bran Crackers: 3 grams fiber per 6 crackers, 110 calories
- Ryvita Dark Rye Whole Grain Crispbread: 3 grams fiber per 2 slices, 70 calories, www.ryvita.com
- Wasa Multi Grain Crispbread: 2 grams fiber per 1 slice, 40 calories

Fruits

- Apples: 5.7 grams fiber per 1 large with peel, 125 calories
- Applesauce—Mott's Organic Unsweetened: 1 gram fiber per ½ cup, 50 calories
- Applesauce—Tree Top: 2 grams fiber per ½ cup, 80 calories
- Avocados: 4.2 grams fiber per ½ cup, 153 calories
- Blackberries: 7.6 grams fiber per 1 cup, 75 calories
- Blueberries: 3.9 grams fiber per 1 cup, 81 calories
- Dates: 3 grams fiber per 5 to 6 pitted (Deglet Noor) dates, 120 calories
- Dried Plums: Sunsweet Bite Size Pitted: 3 grams fiber per 7, 100 calories
- Figs: 3.3 grams fiber per 2 medium, 74 calories
- Kiwi: 5 grams fiber per 2 medium, 93 calories
- Oranges: 3.4 grams fiber per 1 medium, 64 calories
- Papayas: 2.5 grams fiber per 1 cup cubes, 55 calories
- Pears: 4 grams fiber per 1 medium Bartlett, 98 calories
- Persimmons: 6.1 grams fiber per 1 large, 118 calories
- Raisins—Pavich Organic: 2 grams fiber per ¼ cup, 120 calories
- Raisins—Sun-Maid: 2 grams fiber per ¼ cup (1 small box), 130 calories
- Raspberries: 8.4 grams fiber per 1 cup, 60 calories
- Strawberries: 3.5 grams fiber per 1 cup, 46 calories

Juices
- Naked Red Machine: 4 grams fiber (from fruit and flax) per 8 ounces, 160 calories
- Naked Strawberry Banana-C: 3 grams fiber per 8 ounces, 120 calories
- Sunsweet Prune Juice Plus: 3 grams fiber per 8 ounces, 170 calories

Legumes
- Chickpeas: 6.2 grams fiber per ½ cup cooked, 135 calories
- Edensoy Extra Organic Soymilk: 3 grams fiber per 8 ounces, 130 calories
- Green peas: 8.8 grams fiber per 1 cup cooked, 134 calories
- Health Valley Organic Soup—Black Bean (no salt added): 5 grams fiber per 1 cup, 140 calories
- Health Valley Organic Soup—Lentil (no salt added): 8 grams fiber per 1 cup, 110 calories
- Pinto beans: 7.4 grams fiber per ½ cup cooked, 117 calories
- Trader Joe's Dry Roasted Edamame (lightly salted): 4 grams fiber per ¼ cup, 140 calories

Nuts
- Almond Butter—MaraNatha: 3 grams fiber per 2 tablespoons (32 grams), 195 calories
- Almonds (24): 3 grams fiber per 1 ounce, 160 calories
- Hazelnuts (20): 3 grams fiber per 1 ounce, 180 calories
- Pecans (20 halves): 3 grams fiber per 1 ounce, 200 calories
- Pistachios (49): 3 grams fiber per 1 ounce, 160 calories
- Walnuts (14 halves): 2 grams fiber per 1 ounce, 190 calories
- Peanuts (28): 2 grams fiber per 1 ounce, 170 calories

Pizza
- A.C. La Rocco Pizza Company (multiple varieties): 3 to 8 grams fiber per serving
- SuperFoods Kitchen Pizza (multiple varieties): 9 grams fiber per serving

Vegetables
- Asparagus: 2.9 grams fiber per 1 cup cooked, 43 calories
- Broccoli: 4.7 grams fiber per 1 cup cooked, 44 calories
- Butternut squash: 3.5 grams fiber per ½ cup baked, 49 calories
- Cauliflower: 3.3 grams fiber per 1 cup cooked, 29 calories
- Collard greens: 5.3 grams fiber per 1 cup cooked, 49 calories
- Corn: 4.6 grams fiber per 1 cup cooked kernels, 177 calories
- Health Valley Organic Soup—Vegetable (no salt added): 4 grams fiber per 1 cup, 90 calories
- Libby's 100% Canned Pumpkin: 5 grams fiber per ½ cup, 40 calories
- Sweet Potatoes: 3.7 grams per 1 medium (4 ounces), 143 calories
- Swiss chard: 3.7 grams fiber per 1 cup cooked, 35 calories
- Tomatoes: 2.5 grams fiber per 1 medium, 48 calories

LOW-SODIUM FIBER-RICH FOODS

Chips
- Garden of Eatin' Mini Yellow Rounds: 55 mg sodium, 1 gram fiber per 18 chips
- Kettle Brand Chips (unsalted): 0 mg sodium, 2 grams fiber per 1 ounce
- Whole Foods 365 Organic Yellow Corn Tortilla Chips: 80 mg sodium, 4 grams fiber per 16 chips

- Whole Foods 365 Yellow Corn Tortilla Strips: 45 mg sodium, 3 grams fiber per 18 strips

Legumes
- Del Monte Fresh Cut Sweet Peas: 10 mg sodium, 4 grams fiber per ½ cup
- Eden Organic Black Beans (no salt added): 0 mg sodium, 6 grams fiber per ½ cup
- Eden Organic Black Eyed Peas (no salt added): 25 mg sodium, 4 grams fiber per ½ cup
  www.edenfoods.com
- Eden Organic Kidney Beans (no salt added): 15 mg sodium, 10 grams fiber per ½ cup
- Eden Organic Pinto Beans (no salt added): 5 mg sodium, 6 grams fiber per ½ cup
- Health Valley Chunky Chili (no salt added): 75 mg sodium, 10 grams fiber per 1 cup
  www.healthvalley.com
- Ralph's Green Beans Cut (no salt added): 15 mg sodium, 2 grams fiber per ½ cup
- Ralph's Sweet Peas (no salt added): 15 mg sodium, 3 grams fiber per ½ cup
  www.interamericanproducts.com

Low-Sodium Whole Grain Foods
- Arrowhead Mills Organic Oat Bran Pancake and Waffle Mix: 75 mg sodium, 6 grams fiber per ¼ cup
  www.arrowheadmills.com
- Bob's Red Mill Whole Ground Flaxseed Meal: 0 mg sodium, 4 grams fiber per 2 tablespoons
  www.bobsredmill.com
- Breadshop Granola Crunchy Oat Bran with Almonds and Raisins: 0 mg sodium, 4 grams fiber per ½ cup
- Country Choice Organic Irish Style Steel Cut Oats: 0 mg sodium, 4 grams fiber per ¼ cup
  www.countrychoiceorganic.com
- Familia Swiss Muesli: 0 mg sodium, 4 grams fiber per ½ cup
  www.bio-familia.com

- Food for Life Sprouted Grain Ezekiel 4:9 Bread (low sodium): 0 mg sodium, 3 grams fiber per slice
- Garden of Eatin' Blue or Yellow Corn Taco Shells: 5 mg sodium, 1 gram fiber per 2 taco shells www.gardenofeatin.com
- Julian Bakery Cinnamon Almond Raisin Bread: 75 mg sodium, 12 grams fiber per slice www.julianbakery.com
- Kashi Go Lean Cereal: 85 mg sodium, 10 grams fiber per ¾ cup, www.kashi.com
- Kashi Heart to Heart: 90 mg sodium, 5 grams fiber per ¾ cup
- Kashi TLC Tasty Little Chewies Peanut/Peanut Butter, 90 mg sodium, 4 grams fiber per 1 bar
- Trail Mix, 105 mg sodium, 4 grams fiber per 1 bar
- Kretschmer Toasted Wheat Germ: 0 mg sodium, 2 grams fiber per 2 tablespoons www.kretschmer.com
- Post Shredded Wheat and Bran: 0 mg sodium, 8 grams fiber per 1¼ cup www.kraftfoods.com
- Quaker Oat Bran: 0 mg sodium, 6 grams fiber per ½ cup
- Ralph's Whole Wheat Rotini: 0 mg sodium, 5 grams fiber per ¾ cup
- Ronzoni Healthy Harvest 7 Grain Blend Pasta: 0 mg sodium, 5 grams fiber per 2 ounces www.ronzonihealthyharvest.com
- Ronzoni Healthy Harvest Whole Wheat Blend Pasta: 0 mg sodium, 6 grams fiber per 2 ounces
- Whole Foods 365 Organic Whole Wheat Shells: 9 mg sodium, 5 grams fiber per ¾ cup
- Vogel's Soy and Flaxseed Bread: 105 mg sodium, 5 grams fiber per slice 818-761-2892

Tomato Products
- Del Monte Diced Tomatoes (no salt added): 50 mg sodium, 2 grams fiber per ½ cup www.delmonte.com
- Private (PS) Selection (Kroger's) Organic Tomato Paste: 20 mg sodium, 1 gram fiber per 2 tablespoons
- Ralph's Peeled Tomatoes (diced, no salt added): 20 mg sodium, 1 gram fiber per ½ cup
- Ralph's Peeled Tomatoes (whole, no salt added): 20 mg sodium, 1 gram fiber per ½ cup
- Ralph's Tomato Sauce (no salt added): 40 mg sodium, 1 gram fiber per ½ cup
- S&W Ready-Cut Tomatoes (diced, no salt added): 50 mg sodium, 2 grams fiber per ½ cup www.swfinefoods.com

Trail Mix/Snack Foods
- Bear Naked Organic Trail Mix: 0 mg sodium, 2 grams fiber per ¼ cup, 866-374-4442
- Orville Redenbacher's Original Gourmet Popping Corn: 0 mg sodium, 6 grams fiber per 3 tablespoons unpopped

Vegetables
- Del Monte Fresh Cut Whole Kernel Corn (no salt added): 10 mg sodium, 3 grams fiber per ½ cup
- Ralph's Carrots (sliced, no salt added): 55 mg sodium, 2 grams fiber per ½ cup
- Ralph's Mixed Vegetables (no salt added): 25 mg sodium, 1 gram fiber per ½ cup

SUPERFOOD/SIDEKICK SOURCES OF CHOLINE AND BETAINE

Betaine Sources (USDA Database)	Milligrams per 100 mg of food
Baked Products	
Crackers (whole wheat)	212
Graham crackers	194
Bread (whole wheat)	180
Breakfast Cereals	
Wheat germ (toasted)	1396
Kellogg's All-Bran	360
Uncle Sam Cereal	248
Post Shredded Wheat	158
Cereal Grains	
Wheat bran	1507
Wheat (bulgar, cooked)	83
Barley malt flour	66
Oat bran	36
Brown rice	.5
Dairy and Eggs	
Nonfat milk	2.0
Egg yolk (raw)	.9
Mozzarella	.7
Fish and Shellfish	
Shrimp (canned)	33
Tilapia (baked)	26
Crab (blue, canned)	13
Cod (Atlantic, cooked)	10
Tuna (light, canned in water)	3
Fruit	
Raspberries	.8
Avocados	.7
Figs (dried)	.7

Kiwis	.5
Dates (Deglet Noor)	.4
Raisins (seedless)	.3
Watermelon	.3
Strawberries	.2
Blueberries	.2
Cranberries	.2

Legumes

Soy burger	5
Soymilk	.8
Peanuts (raw)	.6
Tofu	.4
Pinto beans	.4

Nuts and Seeds

Cashews	11
Pistachios	.9
Pecans	.7
Almonds	.5
Walnuts	.5
Hazelnuts	.4
Pine nuts	.4
Sesame seeds	.4

Spices and Herbs

Curry powder	28.8
Basil (dried)	16.1
Oregano (dried)	9.8
Pepper (black)	8.9
Garlic powder	6.1
Cinnamon (ground)	3.9

Vegetables

Spinach (frozen whole leaf, cooked)	809
Spinach (frozen chopped, cooked)	726
Spinach (frozen chopped)	675
Beets (raw)	128
Sweet potatoes (cooked)	35
Mushrooms (raw)	11

(continued)

Asparagus (cooked)	.9
Cabbage (raw)	.4
Carrots (raw)	.4
Corn (yellow, kernels)	.2
Ketchup	.2

A daily intake value for betaine has not been established.

Choline Sources (USDA Database)	**Milligrams**
Eggs (1)	110
Cod (4 ounces)	95
Shrimp (4 ounces)	92
Navy beans (1 cup cooked)	82
Salmon (4 ounces)	74
Brussels sprouts (1 cup cooked)	64
Broccoli (1 cup cooked)	63
Pinto beans (1 cup cooked)	62
Kidney beans (1 cup cooked)	60
Cauliflower (1 cup cooked)	49
Asparagus (1 cup cooked)	47
Spinach (1 cup cooked)	45
Green peas (1 cup cooked)	44
Corn (1 cup cooked)	36
Spinach (1 cup frozen, cooked)	36
Buckwheat (1 cup cooked)	34
Tofu (4 ounces)	32
Cabbage (1 cup cooked)	30
Winter squash (1 cup cooked)	22
Cashews (¼ cup)	21
Avocados (1 cup)	21
Peanuts (¼ cup)	19
Almonds (¼ cup)	19

The Institute of Medicine National Academy of Sciences recommendations for choline:

Men 14 years and older	550 mg
Women 14 to 18 years	400 mg
Women 19 years and older	425 mg

Pregnant women	450 mg
Lactating women	550 mg

SUPERFOOD SOURCES OF POTASSIUM

New U.S. government guidelines recommend a daily intake of 4700 milligrams of potassium. My own Super-Health "gene-friendly" recommendation is that you aim for 8000 milligrams a day of potassium. The following list of potassium-rich foods should help you achieve this important goal.

Food Source	Serving Size	Mg of Potassium
Swiss chard	1 cup cooked	960 mg
Sweet potatoes	1 cup cooked	950 mg
Potatoes	1 medium baked	926 mg
Spinach	1 cup cooked	838 mg
Papayas	1 medium	781 mg
Evolution Incredible Vegetable Juice	8 ounces	780 mg
Clams	6 cooked	705 mg
Evolution Organic Carrot Juice	1 cup	640 mg
Citrus C Odwalla C Monster	1 cup	640 mg
Naked Just Carrot Juice	1 cup	620 mg
Butternut squash	1 cup cooked	582 mg
Whole Foods 365 Organic Soymilk	8 ounces	560 mg
Figs (dried)	4 large	541 mg
Sunsweet Prune Juice	1 cup	540 mg
R.W. Knudsen Very Veggie Vegetable Cocktail (low sodium)	1 cup	520 mg

(continued)

Food Source	Serving Size	Mg of Potassium
Libby's Canned Pumpkin	1 cup	505 mg
Broccoli	1 cup cooked	505 mg
Brussels sprouts	1 cup cooked	495 mg
Collard greens	1 cup cooked	494 mg
Cantaloupe	1 cup	494 mg
Naked Juice Strawberry Banana-C	1 cup	480 mg
Kashi Go Lean High Protein and High Fiber Cereal	1 cup	480 mg
Lima beans	½ cup cooked	478 mg
Alta Dena Nonfat Yogurt (fruit on the bottom)	1 cup	475 mg
Lentils	½ cup cooked	475 mg
Naked Juice Just O-J	8 ounces	470 mg
Oysters	6 medium	453 mg
Tropicana 100% Orange Juice	8 ounces	448 mg
R.W. Knudsen Just Pomegranate Juice	8 ounces	440 mg
Edensoy Extra Organic Soymilk	1 cup	440 mg
Avocados	½ Hass avocado	439 mg
POM Wonderful 100%	8 ounces	430 mg
Bananas	1 medium	422 mg
Evolution Organic Tangerine Juice	8 ounces	400 mg
Carrots	1 cup cooked	394 mg
POM Wonderful 100% Pomegranate Cherry Juice	8 ounces	390 mg
Salmon (wild coho)	3 ounces	369 mg
Dried plums (prunes)	6 uncooked	366 mg

Food Source	Serving Size	Mg of Potassium
Trader Joe's Unfiltered Concord Grape Juice	8 ounces	350 mg
Celery	1 cup	344 mg
Oats	½ cup cooked	335 mg
Spinach	2 cups raw	334 mg
Romaine lettuce	2 cups raw	325 mg
Tomato paste	2 tablespoons	324 mg
Dates (Deglet Noor)	6 dates	324 mg
Naked Juice Power C	8 ounces	320 mg
Wild salmon (canned)	3 ounces	320 mg
Raisins	¼ cup	309 mg
Silk Vanilla Soymilk	1 cup	300 mg
Kale	1 cup cooked	296 mg
Pinto beans	½ cup canned	292 mg
Asparagus	1 cup cooked	288 mg
Blackberries	1 cup	282 mg
Kirkland Organic Vanilla Soymilk	8 ounces	280 mg
Kiwis	1 kiwi	253 mg
Strawberries	1 cup	252 mg
Turkey (skinless breast)	3 ounces	248 mg
Apricots (dried)	6 halves	246 mg
Oranges	1 medium	237 mg
Broccoli (cooked)	½ cup	228 mg
Tofu	½ cup	221 mg
Chickpeas (garbanzo beans)	½ cup	207 mg
Almonds	1 ounce	198 mg

(continued)

Food Source	Serving Size	Mg of Potassium
Peanuts	1 ounce	191 mg
Tomatoes (raw)	½ cup	183 mg
Applesauce (unsweetened)	½ cup	183 mg
Flaxseed (ground)	1 tablespoon	164 mg
Figs	1 large (½-inch diameter)	148 mg
Wheat germ	2 tablespoons	134 mg
Walnuts	1 ounce	124 mg
Turmeric	2 teaspoons	115 mg
Nestlé Carnation Evaporated Fat Free Milk	2 tablespoons	110 mg

12

SuperHealth Recipes

❖ Banana Bran Muffins

1¼ cups whole wheat flour
1½ cups oat bran
1 tablespoon baking powder
¼ cup honey
¾ cup plain or vanilla soymilk
1 cup mashed bananas
1 egg
1 cup chopped almonds (optional)
½ teaspoon orange zest (orange peel grated)
¼ cup Smart Balance oil

Preheat the oven to 400°F. Line a 12-muffin tin with paper liners.

In a large bowl, mix the flour, bran, and baking powder. In a separate bowl, mix the honey, soymilk, bananas, egg, orange zest, and oil. Slowly add the flour mixture to the banana mixture. Stir in almonds, if using. Divide the batter among the muffin cups (fill each ¾ full) and bake for 20 minutes, until slightly brown. Cool for 10 minutes in the pan, then remove.

❖ Dr. Steve's Hot Chocolate

1 cup vanilla soymilk
1 teaspoon dark honey
4 tablespoons (about 22 grams) cocoa powder, preferably Dagoda Organic Chocolate Cocoa Powder or Rapunzel Organic Cocoa Powder, or to taste

Mix the soymilk and honey in a mug and microwave for 1 minute. Stir to dissolve the honey, then add cocoa powder and stir to dissolve. Serve immediately.

❖ SuperHealth Spinach Salad

1 cup spinach torn into bite-size pieces
1 cup chopped romaine lettuce
¼ cup shredded red cabbage
½ cup sliced red bell pepper
½ tomato, chopped (or orange, yellow, or green bell pepper)
¼ cup cooked chickpeas (if canned, rinse well—the water they are packed in can be quite salty)
½ cup grated carrot
¼ avocado, cubed
2 tablespoons extra virgin olive oil
1 teaspoon balsamic vinegar

Combine the spinach, lettuce, cabbage, red pepper, tomato, chickpeas, carrot, and avocado in a large bowl. In a separate bowl, whisk together the oil and vinegar. Toss the dressing with the salad just before serving.

If you like, add a sprinkle of ground peppercorns, a handful of your favorite chopped fresh herbs, 1 tablespoon Parmigiano-Reggiano, or 2 tablespoons roasted nuts or seeds.

This quantity is for one person, but you can easily scale up the ingredients to serve more.

❖ Orange-Poppyseed Dressing

½ cup cold-pressed extra virgin olive oil
Zest of ½ orange
Juice of 1 orange
Juice of 1 lemon
2 tablespoons honey
1 tablespoon poppyseeds or toasted sesame seeds

Put all the ingredients in a lidded jar and shake until blended. Refrigerate for at least 2 hours to let the flavors develop. This is a delightful dressing for spinach salad or fruit salad.

❖ Grant's Guacamole

4 ripe avocados
1 tablespoon chili powder
¼ teaspoon garlic powder
1 tablespoon La Victoria Taco Sauce
½ teaspoon lemon juice

Peel the avocados and mash them in a large bowl. Stir in remaining ingredients. Cover with plastic and refrigerate for 30 minutes. Serve immediately.

❖ Torey's Quinoa Delight

1 cup cooked quinoa
2 cups chopped fresh basil
½ cup olive oil
½ cup diced cherry tomatoes
2 tablespoons pesto (store-bought or homemade), or to taste

In a large bowl, mix the ingredients together. If you like, you can garnish with toasted walnuts, pine nuts, almonds, or other nuts of your choice.

❖ Peggy's Wheat Germ Cornbread

1 cup whole wheat flour
2 teaspoons sugar
5 teaspoons baking powder
1 cup wheat germ
1 cup cornmeal
3 eggs
1½ cups milk
¼ cup Smart Balance oil
2 teaspoons honey

Preheat the oven to 375°F and grease a 9-inch loaf pan.
In a large bowl, mix flour, sugar, and baking powder.
Stir in the wheat germ and cornmeal. In a separate
bowl, beat the eggs and milk, then add the oil and
honey. Stir into the flour mixture just to moisten. Trans-
fer to the loaf pan and bake for 40 to 45 minutes, until
knife or toothpick comes out clean. Cool for 10 minutes.

❖ Gunni's Moosh-a-Magulla Vegetable and Salmon Stir-Fry

½ cup extra virgin olive oil
1 large onion, diced
½ cup diced carrots
1 clove garlic, minced
1 orange bell pepper, diced
2 tablespoons Kirkland Organic No-Salt Seasoning
or other no-salt seasoning
1 cup chopped broccoli
1 cup cooked soybeans
2 medium tomatoes, diced
1 cup frozen corn kernels
½ pound wild Alaskan salmon (chopped into medium
pieces)
2 cups chopped kale

In skillet over medium-high heat, combine the oil,
onion, carrots, garlic, bell pepper, and no-salt seasoning.

Stir-fry until the vegetables are lightly browned. Add the broccoli and soybeans and stir-fry for 3 minutes. Reduce heat to low and add the tomatoes, corn, salmon, and kale. Cook for about 7 minutes, stirring occasionally, until the salmon is cooked through. Serve with baked sweet potatoes or brown rice.

You can substitute vegetables of your choice for any of the vegetables.

❖ Turkey Enchiladas

2 tablespoons olive oil
1 large onion, chopped
1 pound ground turkey breast
1 small can (8 ounces) salt-free tomato sauce
2 19-ounce cans La Victoria Enchilada sauce
12 corn tortillas
2 cups shredded low-fat cheddar cheese

Preheat the oven to 375°F. In a large skillet over medium-high heat, heat the oil. Add the onion and sauté until slightly softened, about 3 minutes. Add the ground turkey and cook until browned. In a large bowl, mix together the tomato sauce and enchilada sauce.

Spray the bottom and sides of a large casserole dish with cooking spray. Cover with a layer of tortillas, followed by half the turkey mixture and 1 cup of the cheese, and spread evenly. Pour one-third of the sauce evenly over the top. Add another layer of tortillas, meat, and cheese. Pour one-third of the sauce evenly over this layer, followed by a third layer of tortillas on top. Pour the last third of the sauce evenly over this layer. Bake for 45 minutes, or until hot and bubbly.

❖ Turkey Macaroni

2 tablespoons extra virgin olive oil
1 large onion, diced
½ pound ground turkey breast
1 teaspoon dried basil
1 teaspoon dried oregano
1 teaspoon fresh crushed garlic
1 teaspoon pepper
One 14.5-ounce can no-salt-added diced tomatoes
Two 6-ounce cans organic no-salt-added tomato paste
1 cup water
4 cups cooked whole wheat macaroni pasta

Preheat the oven to 375°F. In a large skillet, heat the oil over medium-high heat. Add the onion, turkey, basil, oregano, garlic, and pepper and cook until the turkey is browned. Turn the heat off and add the diced tomatoes, tomato paste, and water. Mix until well blended. Add the cooked pasta and mix gently. Fold into a glass casserole pan, cover with foil, and bake for 25 to 30 minutes, or until hot and steaming. Serve with Peggy's Wheat Germ Cornbread (page 282).

❖ Turkey Spaghetti

2 tablespoons extra virgin olive oil
1 large onion, chopped
1 pound ground turkey breast
Two 6-ounce cans no-salt-added tomato paste
1 large can (15 ounces) no-salt-added tomato sauce
1 large tomato, diced
1 cup water
2 tablespoons Italian seasoning (salt free)
4 cups cooked organic whole wheat spaghetti

In a large skillet, heat the oil over medium-high heat. Add the onion and ground turkey and cook until the turkey is browned. Add the tomato paste, tomato sauce, diced tomato, and water, then add the Italian seasoning, and bring to a simmer. Serve the sauce over the noodles.

❖ Healthy Oatmeal Cookies

2 sticks Smart Balance 50/50 Butter Blend, softened
2 eggs
1½ cups honey
2 tablespoons ground cinnamon
1½ cups unsweetened applesauce
2½ cups whole wheat flour
1 cup flaxseed meal
1 teaspoon baking soda
1 teaspoon baking powder
2 cups rolled oats
2 cups raisins

Preheat the oven to 375°F and coat a cookie sheet with cooking spray (I use Pam).

In a large bowl, cream the Smart Balance, eggs, honey, and cinnamon. Blend in the applesauce. In a separate bowl, mix the flour, flaxseed meal, baking soda, and baking powder. Add to the Smart Balance mixture and mix well. Blend in the oats and raisins and drop by teaspoonfuls onto the cookie sheet. Bake for 6 to 8 minutes, until slightly brown. Cool for 5 minutes on cookie sheet, then remove.

❖ Mike and Diane's Pumpkin Cookies

1 large (20-ounce) can Libby's 100% Pure Pumpkin
1 egg
½ cup melted Smart Balance 50/50 Butter Blend
¾ cup dark honey
¼ cup ground cinnamon
2 cups whole wheat pastry flour
¾ cup oat bran
1 cup chopped almonds (optional)
1 cup raisins (optional)

Preheat oven to 375°F and lightly grease a cookie sheet with cooking spray.

In a large bowl, mix the pumpkin, egg, Smart Balance, honey, and cinnamon. In a separate bowl, mix the flour and oat bran. Stir the flour mixture into the pumpkin mixture. Fold in the nuts and raisins, if using. Drop by teaspoons onto the cookie sheet. Bake for 15 minutes, until knife or toothpick comes out clean. Cool for 10 minutes.

❖ Marlaina's Pumpkin Pie Smoothie

1 cup Libby's 100% Pure Canned Pumpkin
1 cup lowfat vanilla frozen yogurt
1 cup unsweetened applesauce
2 cups organic vanilla soymilk
1 scoop (30 grams) vanilla whey protein (e.g., Jay Robb Vanilla Whey Protein)
1 tablespoon ground cinnamon
2 cups ice cubes

Put all the ingredients into a blender and blend on high speed until smooth.

13

Weekly Food and Exercise Planners and Shopping Lists

Week 1: Omega-3 and Resveratrol (RES) Daily Food Planner

	Food Suggestion	Daily Servings
Day 1	Wild salmon	3–4 ounces (1 deck of cards)
	Spinach	1 cup steamed (1 baseball)
	Walnuts	1 handful (1 layer on your palm)
	Soymilk	2 cups (16 ounces)
	Flaxseed	2 tablespoons ground (1 shot glass)
	Blueberries (RES)	1 cup (1 baseball)
Day 2	DHA eggs	2 eggs
	Spinach	2 cups raw (2 baseballs)
	Pecans	1 handful (1 layer on your palm)
	Tofu	½ cup raw tofu (½ baseball)
	Wheat germ	2 tablespoons (1 shot glass)
	Soybean oil	2 tablespoons (1 shot glass)
	Purple grape juice (RES)	½ cup (4 ounces)
Day 3	Alaskan halibut	3–4 ounces (1 deck of cards)
	Spinach	1 cup steamed (1 baseball)
	Soymilk	2 cups (16 ounces)
	Flaxseed	2 tablespoons ground (1 shot glass)
		(continued)

Day 3 (*cont.*)	Peanut butter (RES)	2 tablespoons (1 walnut in a shell)
Day 4	Pecans	1 handful (1 layer on your palm)
	Soymilk	2 cups (16 ounces)
	Wheat germ	2 tablespoons (1 shot glass)
	Red wine (RES)	One 4.5-ounce glass
Day 5	DHA eggs	2 eggs
	Collard greens	1 cup steamed (1 baseball)
	Pumpkin seeds	1 handful (1 layer on your palm)
	Tofu	½ cup raw tofu (½ baseball)
	Flaxseed	2 tablespoons ground (1 shot glass)
	Blueberries (RES)	1 cup (1 baseball)
Day 6	Canned chunk light tuna	3–4 ounces (1 deck of cards)
	Soy nuts	1 handful (1 layer on your palm)
	Flaxseed	2 tablespoons ground (1 shot glass)
	Soybean oil	1 tablespoon (½ shot glass)
	Peanuts (RES)	1 handful (1 layer on your palm)
Day 7	DHA eggs	2 eggs
	Spinach	2 cups raw (2 baseballs)
	Walnuts	1 handful (1 layer on your palm)
	Soymilk	2 cups (16 ounces)
	Wheat germ	2 tablespoons (1 shot glass)
	Canola oil	1 tablespoon (½ shot glass)
	Cranberry juice (RES)	½ cup (4 ounces)

Week 1: Control Your Genes Shopping List
(Always look for no-salt-added or low-sodium products.)

Wild salmon + Sidekicks
Fresh spinach + Sidekicks
Fresh purple grapes
Fresh blueberries
Fresh broccoli
Red wine

Bottled Juice

- Columbia Gorge Certified Organic Juices (multiple flavors) www.CoGoJuice.com
- Kedem Concord 100% Pure Grape Juice
- Kirkland Cranberry-Grape 100% Juice Blend
- Kirkland 100% Grape Juice
- Minute Maid 100% Pure Grape Juice
- Mountain Sun Pure Cranberry Juice (100% pure unsweetened cranberry juice is tart, so mix it with another, sweeter 100% pure fruit juice)
- Ocean Spray Premium 100% Cranberry Juice
- R.W. Knudsen Family Just Concord
- R.W. Knudsen Family Organic Cranberry Juice
- Trader Joe's All-Natural Triple Berry Juice 100% Juice Blend from Pomegranates, Blueberries, and Cranberries
- Trader Joe's 100% Unfiltered Concord Grape Juice
- Walnut Acres Certified Organic Concord Grape Juice
- Walnut Acres Certified Organic Wild Cranberry Juice
- Welch's 100% Grape Juice

Canned Albacore Tuna

- Bumble Bee Solid White Albacore Tuna in Water
- Chicken of the Sea Chunk Light Tuna in Canola Oil
- Chicken of the Sea Low-Sodium Chunk White Albacore Tuna
- Kirkland Solid White Albacore Tuna Packed in Water
- StarKist Solid White Albacore Tuna in Water
- Trader Joe's White Solid Albacore Tuna (reduced sodium)

Canned Clams and Crab
- Sea Watch Chopped Sea Clams
- Trader Joe's Chopped Sea Clams
- Trader Joe's Crab Meat

Canned Salmon
- Bumble Bee Alaskan Pink Salmon
- Bumble Bee Alaskan Sockeye Red Salmon
- Chicken of the Sea Pink Salmon
- Crown Prince Fancy Alaskan Pink Salmon (low sodium) www.crownprince.com
- Libby's Red Salmon
- Trader Joe's Alaskan Pink Salmon
- Trader Joe's Red Salmon
- Vital Choice Wild Red Sockeye Salmon (no sodium added)

Frozen Fish
- High Liner Atlantic Cod Fillets
- Kauai Shrimp Fresh Island Fish www.freshislandfish.com
- Ocean Beauty Wild Alaskan Salmon
- Omstead Fresh Water Cleaned Smelt 519-825-7144
- Vital Choice Alaskan Fish Fillets (multiple varieties)
- Whole Foods Market wild sockeye salmon, scallops, shrimp, yellowfin tuna steaks, wild Alaskan cod fillets

Ground Flaxseed/Wheat Germ
- Bob's Red Mill Whole Ground Flaxseed
- Kretschmer Original Toasted Wheat Germ

Nuts and Seeds
- Ann's House of Nuts Unsalted Dry-Roasted Peanuts
- Elizabeth's Natural No-Salt Roasted in Shell Pumpkin Seeds.

- Elizabeth's Natural Pecans
- Elizabeth's Natural Raw Almonds
- Elizabeth's Natural Raw Cashews
- Elizabeth's Natural Raw Hulled Sunflower Seeds
- Elizabeth's Natural Walnuts
- Hoody's Classic Roast Peanuts (Original Nut House Brand)
- Kirkland Almonds
- Kirkland Pecan Halves
- Kirkland Walnuts
- Old Tyme Peanuts (no salt or oil)

- Planters Unsalted Peanuts
- Trader Joe's California Premium Walnut Halves
- Trader Joe's California Walnut Halves and Pieces
- Trader Joe's Dry Roasted and Unsalted Pistachios
- Trader Joe's Raw Pecan Pieces
- Trader Joe's Raw Sunflower Seeds
- Trader Joe's Roasted and Unsalted Whole Cashews

Peanut Butter

- Arrowhead Mills Crunchy Valencia Peanut Butter
- Arrowhead Mills 100% Valencia Peanut Butter

- Laura Scudder's Old Fashioned Peanut Butter (no salt added)

Sardines

- Beach Cliff Sardines in Soybean Oil
- Bela Olhão Portugal Lightly Smoked Sardines in Olive Oil
- Crown Prince One Layer Brisling Sardines in Oil
- Crown Prince Skinless and Boneless Sardines in Olive Oil

- King Oscar Extra Small Sardines in Purest Virgin Olive Oil
- Yankee Clipper Lightly Smoked Sardines in Lemon Sauce
- Yankee Clipper Lightly Smoked Sardines in Tomato Sauce

Soy Products

- Eden Organic Soymilk
- Kirkland (Costco) Soymilk
- Nasoya Organic Tofu www.nasoya.com
- Pacific Soymilk
- Revival Soy Nuts (unsalted) www.revivalsoy.com
- Silk Soymilk
- Soy Boy Organic Tofu www.soyboy.com
- Soy Dream Soymilk
- Super Soynuts (unsalted) www.soynuts.com
- Trader Joe's Soymilk
- VitaSoy Soymilk
- WestSoy Soymilk
- Whole Foods 365 Everyday Value Organic Tofu

Week 2: Green Eating Daily Food Planner

	Food Suggestion	Daily Servings
Day 1	Soy nuts	¼ cup (1 layer on your palm)
	Apple	1 medium (1 baseball)
	Broccoli sprouts	2 cups (2 baseballs)
	Onion	¼ medium (¼ baseball)
	Garlic	To taste
	Spices	To taste
	Tea	4 cups
Day 2	Tofu	½ cup raw tofu (½ baseball)
	Apple	1 medium (1 baseball)
	Brussels sprouts (raw or cooked)	2 cups (2 baseballs) raw or cooked
	Chives	¼ cup (¼ baseball)
	Garlic	To taste
	Spices	To taste
	Tea	4 cups
Day 3	Edamame	1 cup (1 baseball)
	Pear	1 medium (1 baseball)
	Red cabbage (raw or cooked)	1–2 cups (1–2 baseballs) raw or ½ cup cooked (½ baseball)
	Leeks (raw or cooked)	¼ cup (¼ baseball) raw or cooked
	Garlic	To taste

	Food Suggestion	**Daily Servings**
	Spices	To taste
	Tea	4 cups
Day 4	Soy yogurt	One 6-ounce container
	Apple	1 medium (1 baseball)
	Kale	2 cups (2 baseballs)
	Onion	¼ medium (¼ baseball)
	Garlic	To taste
	Spices	To taste
	Tea	4 cups
Day 5	Soymilk	2 cups (16 ounces)
	Apple	1 medium (1 baseball)
	Broccoli (raw or cooked)	2 cups (2 baseballs) raw or ½ cup cooked (½ baseball)
	Chives	¼ cup (¼ baseball)
	Garlic	To taste
	Spices	To taste
	Tea	4 cups
Day 6	Tempeh	½ cup (½ baseball)
	Pear	1 medium (1 baseball)
	Collard greens	2 cups (2 baseballs)
	Scallions	¼ cup (¼ baseball)
	Garlic	To taste
	Spices	To taste
	Tea	4 cups
Day 7	Tofu	½ cup raw tofu (½ baseball)
	Apple	1 medium (1 baseball)
	Broccoli sprouts	2 cups (2 baseballs)
	Onion	¼ medium (¼ baseball)
	Garlic	To taste
	Spices	To taste
	Tea	4 cups

Week 2: Become an Environmentalist Shopping List

*(Always look for no-salt-added or
low-sodium products.)*

Fresh onions, garlic + Sidekicks
Fresh broccoli + Sidekicks
Fresh apples

Black Tea
- Bigelow Tea
- Celestial Seasonings Tea
- Choice Organic Tea
- Lipton Tea
- Numi Organic Tea
- Stash Tea
- Tazo Tea
- Twinings Tea
- Yogi Tea

Green Cleaning Products
- Arm & Hammer
  Baking Soda
  www.armhammer.com
- Bio-Kleen
  www.biokleen.com
- Dr. Bronner
  www.drbronner.com
- Earth Friendly
  www.ecos.com
- Ecover
  www.ecover.com
- Mrs. Meyers
  www.mrsmeyers.com
- Seventh Generation
  www.seventhgen.com
- Simple Green
  www.simplegreen.com

Green Tea
- Bigelow Green Tea:
  plain, peach, mint,
  lemon, variety pack
- Celestial Seasonings
  Green: Authentic,
  Honey Lemon Ginseng
- Choice Organic Tea
- Good Earth Green Tea
  Blend with Lemongrass
- Lipton Green Tea
- Mighty Leaf Organic
  Green Teas: Tropical
  Green, Hojicha
- Numi Organic Green
  Tea
- Salada 100% Green
  Tea
- Stash Chai Green Tea
- Tazo China Green Tips,
  Zen
- Twinings Green
- Yogi Green Tea

Organic Fertilizer/Pesticides

- Bio Flora Dry Crumbles
  www.bioflora.com
- Dr. Bronner's Peppermint Castille Soap
  www.drbronner.com
- Dr. Earth Fruit and Vegetable Insect Spray
  www.drearth.com
- Dr. Earth House and Garden Plants Insect Spray
- Dr. Earth Organic Fruit Tree, Flower Garden, or Tomato, Vegetable, and Herb Fertilizers
- E.B. Stone organic mulch and fertilizer
  www.ebstone.org
- Garden Defense Multi-Purpose Spray
  www.arbico-organics.com

Rooibos Tea

- Choice Organic Rooibos Red Bush Tea
  www.choiceorganics.com

Soymilk

- Eden Organic Soymilk
- Kirkland (Costco) Soymilk
- Pacific Soymilk
- Silk Soymilk
- Soy Dream Soymilk
- Trader Joe's Soymilk
- VitaSoy Soymilk
- WestSoy Soymilk
- Wild Wood Organics Organic Real Vanilla Soymilk
  www.wildwoodfoods.com

Soy Products

- Nasoya Organic Tofu
  www.nasoya.com
- Seapoint Farms Dry Roasted Edamame
  www.seapointfarms.com
- Seapoint Farms Frozen Shelled Edamame
- Silk Live Soy Yogurt
  www.silksoymilk.com
- Soy Boy 5 Grain Tempeh
- Soy Boy Organic Tempeh
- Soy Boy Organic Tofu
  www.soyboy.com

- Stonyfield O'Soy Yogurt
www.stonyfield.com
- Whole Foods 365 Everyday Value Organic Tofu

- WholeSoy Yogurt
www.wholesoyco.com

Spices and Seasonings

- Kirkland Organic No Salt Seasoning
- Lizzie's Kitchen Herbs de Provence, Garden Vegetable
- McCormick Salt Free All Purpose, Salt Free It's a Dilly
- Mrs. Dash—any of the nine Seasoning Blends or four Grilling Blends
- Spice Hunter Organic Salt Free Italian Seasoning, Salt-Free Herbs de Provence, Salt Free Barbecue Grill Spice, Red Pepper (ground cayenne), Arrowroot (ground)

- Spice Islands Salt Free Seasoning Citrus Herbs, Mediterranean Seasoning, Fines Herbes, Garlic Herb Blend, Rosemary Garlic Blend
- Various other spices, including: cinnamon, pumpkin pie spice, oregano, thyme, turmeric, garlic, cumin, parsley, sage, rosemary, mint, mustard, dill, orange peel
- Vital Choice organic spices
www.vitalchoice.com

Week 3: Watch Your Waistline Weekly Food Planner

	Food Suggestion	Daily Servings
Day 1	Unsweetened applesauce	½ cup (½ baseball)
	Ground flaxseed	2 tablespoons (1 shot glass)
	Yogurt	1 cup (1 baseball)
	Carrots	½ cup (½ baseball)
	Tomato	1 medium (1 baseball)
	Lentils (cooked)	½ cup (½ baseball)
	Buckwheat honey	1 to 2 tablespoons (½ to 1 shot glass)
	EVOO	2 tablespoons (1 shot glass)

	Food Suggestion	**Daily Servings**
Day 2	Avocado	½ cup (½ baseball)
	Wheat bran	2 tablespoons (1 shot glass)
	Yogurt (soy)	1 cup (1 baseball)
	Pumpkin	½ cup (½ baseball)
	Tomato paste	2 tablespoons (1 shot glass)
	Chickpeas	½ cup (½ baseball)
	Buckwheat honey	1 to 2 tablespoons (½ to 1 shot glass)
	EVOO	2 tablespoons (1 shot glass)
Day 3	Blueberries	1 cup (1 baseball)
	Whole grain bread	2 slices
	Yogurt	1 cup (1 baseball)
	Sweet potato	½ cup (½ baseball)
	Pink grapefruit	½ grapefruit
	String beans	1 cup (1 baseball)
	Buckwheat honey	1 to 2 tablespoons (½ to 1 shot glass)
	EVOO	2 tablespoons (1 shot glass)
Day 4	Orange	1 medium (1 baseball)
	Bran cereal	1 cup (1 baseball)
	Carrots	½ cup (½ baseball)
	Tomato	1 medium (1 baseball)
	EVOO	2 tablespoons (1 shot glass)
Day 5	Pear	1 medium (1 baseball)
	Quinoa (cooked)	½ cup (½ baseball)
	Yogurt (soy)	1 cup (1 baseball)
	Butternut squash	½ cup (½ baseball)
	Tomato	1 medium (1 baseball)
	Kidney beans (cooked)	½ cup (½ baseball)
	Buckwheat honey	1 to 2 tablespoons (½ to 1 shot glass)
	EVOO	2 tablespoons (1 shot glass)
Day 6	Strawberries	1 cup (1 baseball)
	Brown rice (cooked)	½ cup (½ baseball)
	Yogurt	1 cup (1 baseball)
	Orange bell pepper	½ cup (½ baseball)
	Watermelon	1 cup cubed (1 baseball)

(continued)

	Food Suggestion	Daily Servings
Day 6 (*cont.*)	Buckwheat honey	1 to 2 tablespoons (½ to 1 shot glass)
	EVOO	2 tablespoons (1 shot glass)
Day 7	Nectarine	1 medium (1 baseball)
	Ground flaxseed	2 tablespoons (1 shot glass)
	Pumpkin	½ cup (½ baseball)
	Tomato	1 medium (1 baseball)
	Green peas	½ cup (½ baseball)
	Buckwheat honey	1 to 2 tablespoons (½ to 1 shot glass)
	EVOO	2 tablespoons (1 shot glass)

Week 3: Watch Your Waistline Daily Exercise Planner

	Exercise	Set Reminders
Day 1	Walk	15 minutes
	Power Stairs	5 minutes
	Heel to Fanny	3 sets of 10
	Isometric Curl	10 times with both arms
	Isometric Extension	10 times with both arms
	Ball Squeeze	10 times
Day 2	Walk	15 minutes
	Heel to Fanny	3 sets of 10
	Sit-up/Crunch	3 sets of 10
	Isometric Curl	10 times with both arms
	Isometric Extension	10 times with both arms
Day 3	Walk	15 minutes
	Power Stairs	5 minutes
	Ball Squeeze	10 times
	Stand Up/Sit Down/Wall Sit	Unlimited times
Day 4	Walk	15 minutes
	Heel to Fanny	3 sets of 10
	Sit-up/Crunch	3 sets of 10
	Isometric Curl	10 times with both arms
	Isometric Extension	10 times with both arms
	Ball Squeeze	10 times
	Stand Up/Sit Down/Wall Sit	Unlimited times

	Exercise	Set Reminders
Day 5	Walk	15 minutes
	Power Stairs	5 minutes
	Isometric Curl	10 times with both arms
	Isometric Extension	10 times with both arms
	Ball Squeeze	10 times
Day 6	Walk	15 minutes
	Heel to Fanny	3 sets of 10
	Sit-up/Crunch	3 sets of 10
	Ball Squeeze	10 times
	Stand Up/Sit Down/Wall Sit	Unlimited times
Day 7	Walk	15 minutes
	Power Stairs	5 minutes
	Isometric Curl	10 times with both arms
	Isometric Extension	10 times with both arms

Week 3: Watch Your Waistline Shopping List

*(Always look for no-salt-added or
low-sodium products.)*

Fresh fruit
Fresh tomatoes + Sidekicks
Fresh pumpkin + Sidekicks

Applesauce
- Santa Cruz Organic Applesauce
  www.scojuice.com

Bread
- Arnold's 100% Whole
  Wheat 9 Grain
  Bread
- The Baker Honey
  Cinnamon Raisin
  Bread
  www.the-baker.com
- The Baker 9-Grain
  Whole Wheat Bread
- The Baker Seeded
  Whole Wheat Bread
- The Baker 7-Grain
  Sourdough Whole
  Wheat Bread

- The Baker Whole Grain Rye
- Ezekiel 4:9 Bread—Sprouted Grain (low sodium)
- Food for Life Sprouted Wheat Burger Buns www.foodforlife.com
- Julian Bakery 12-Grain Sandwich Bread www.julianbakery.com
- Milton's Healthy Multi-Grain Bread www.miltonsbaking.com
- Natural Ovens Bakery Breads www.naturalovens.com
- Pepperidge Farm 9 Grain Natural 100% Whole Grain Bread
- Roman Meal 100% Whole Wheat Bread
- Rudi's Organic Bakery Honey Sweet Whole Wheat Bread www.rudisbakery.com
- Sara Lee 100% Whole Wheat Bread

Canned Pumpkin
- Libby's 100% Pure Pumpkin

Canned Tomato Products
- Classico DiNapoli Spicy Red Pepper Pasta Sauce
- Classico DiNapoli Tomato and Basil Pasta Sauce
- Colavita 100% Natural Marinara Sauce www.colavita.com
- Del Monte Diced Tomatoes (no salt added)
- Emeril's Roasted Red Pepper Pasta Sauce
- Hunt's Tomato Sauce (no salt added)
- Muir Glen Organic Chunky Tomato and Herb Pasta Sauce
- Muir Glen Organic Chunky Tomato Sauce www.muirglen.com
- Muir Glen Organic Crushed Tomatoes with Basil
- Muir Glen Organic Ground Peeled Tomatoes
- Muir Glen Organic Tomato Paste
- Muir Glen Organic Tomato Puree

- Muir Glen Organic Whole Peeled Tomatoes
- Private Selection (PS) Organic Tomato Paste (Kroger's)
- Ralph's Peeled Tomatoes (diced, no salt added)
- Ralph's Peeled Tomatoes (whole, no salt added)
- Ralph's Tomato Sauce (no salt added)
- S&W Petite-Cut Diced Tomatoes in Rich, Thick Juice
- S&W Ready-Cut Tomatoes (diced, no salt added)
- Walnut Acres Organic Zesty Basil Pasta Sauce www.walnutacres.com

Cold Cereal

- Alpen Naturally Delicious Swiss Style Cereal (low fat)
- Alpen Swiss Style Cereal (no added sugar or salt)
- Arrowhead Mills Organic Spelt Flakes
- Back to Nature Granola www.organicmilling.com
- Back to Nature Ultra Flax
- Barbara's Bite Size Shredded Oats Crunchy Wholegrain Cereal www.barbarasbakery.com
- Barbara's Grain Shop High Fiber Cereal
- Bob's Red Mill Natural Raw Wheat Germ
- Bob's Red Mill Whole Ground Flaxseed Meal
- Breadshop's Cranberry Crunch Muesli
- Breadshop's Granola Crunchy Oat Bran with Almonds and Raisins
- Cheerios
- Familia Low-Fat Granola
- Familia No Added Sugar Swiss Muesli
- Familia Original Recipe Muesli
- Galaxy Granola Radically Raspberry www.galaxygranola.com
- Health Valley Organic Amaranth Flakes
- Health Valley Organic Multigrain Flakes
- Health Valley Organic Oat Bran Flakes
- Health Valley Organic Oat Bran O's
- Kashi Go Lean Good Friends Cereal
- Kashi Go Lean Protein and High Fiber Cereal
- Kashi Go Lean Seven Whole Grains and Sesame
- Kellogg's Complete Oat Bran Flakes

- Kellogg's Complete Wheat Bran Flakes
- Kretschmer Toasted Wheat Germ
- Nature's Path Heritage O's
- Nature's Path Organic Blueberry Muesli
- Nature's Path Organic Optimum Power Breakfast Cereal— Flax-Soy-Blueberry
- Organic Fiber 7 Multigrain Flakes

- Post Grape-Nuts Flakes
- Post Shredded Wheat 'N Bran
- Trader Joe's Organic Golden Flax Cereal
- Uncle Sam Cereal— Toasted Whole Grain Wheat Flakes with Crispy Whole Flaxseed
- Weetabix Organic Cereal

Cooked Cereal

- Bob's Red Mill 7 Grain Hot Cereal www.bobsredmill.com
- Hodgson Mill Natural Oat Bran All Hot Cereal
- McCann's Instant Irish Oatmeal (regular flavor)
- McCann's Quick Cooking Irish Oatmeal
- McCann's Steel Cut Irish Oatmeal
- Mother's 100% Natural Rolled Oats
- Mother's 100% Natural Whole Grain Barley

- Quaker Instant Oatmeal (original)
- Quaker Oat Bran Hot Cereal
- Quaker Old-Fashioned Oats
- Quaker Quick Oats
- Silver Palate Thick and Rough Oatmeal
- Stone-Buhr 7 Grain Cereal www.s-bcereals.com
- Stone-Buhr 4 Grain Cereal Mates
- Wheatena Toasted Wheat Cereal

Honey

- Gourmet Honey Store Buckwheat Honey www.gourmethoneystore .com

- Honey Gardens Apitherapy Raw Honey www.honeygardens.com

- Miller's Select
Honey—Buckwheat
www.millershoney
.com

- Topanga Quality
Honey—Buckwheat
www.rawunfileredhoney
.com

Whole Grains

- Fantastic Organic
Whole Wheat Couscous
www.fantasticfoods.com
- Lundberg Family
Farms Organic Long
Grain Brown Rice
www.lundberg.com
- Lundberg Family
Farms Organic Short
Grain Brown Rice
- Lundberg Family
Farms Organic Wild
Rice Blend
- Ralph's Whole Wheat
Whole Grain Rotini
- Ronzoni Healthy
Harvest 7 Grain Pasta

- Ronzoni Healthy
Harvest Whole Wheat
Blend Pasta
- Texmati Long Grain
American Basmati
Brown Rice
- Trader Joe's Basmati
Rice Medley
- Trader Joe's Brown
Rice Medley
- Trader Joe's California
Brown Aromatic Rice
- Trader Joe's Red Rice
- Trader Joe's Rice
Trilogy

Yogurt

- Alta Dena Nonfat
Yogurt (multiple
flavors)
www.altadenadairy.com
- Cascade Fresh Fat Free
Yogurt (multiple
flavors)
www.cascadefresh.com
- Colombo Nonfat Yogurt
(multiple flavors)
- Continental Non Fat
Yogurt (multiple flavors)
- DanActive Immunity
Probiotic Dairy Drink

- Horizon Organic Fat
Free Yogurt (multiple
flavors)
- Stonyfield Farm Nonfat
Yogurt (multiple
flavors)
- Stonyfield Farm
Organic Yogurt
Smoothie (multiple
flavors)
- Sustenex supplements
- Trader Joe's French
Village Low Fat/Nonfat
Yogurt (multiple flavors)

Week 4: Control Inflammation Daily Food Planner

	Food Suggestion	**Daily Servings**
Day 1	Wild salmon	3–4 ounces (1 deck of cards)
	Flaxseed	2 tablespoons ground (1 shot glass)
	Garlic	To taste
	EVOO	2 tablespoons (1 shot glass)
Day 2	Skinless turkey breast	3–4 ounces (1 deck of cards)
	Brown rice	½ cup (½ baseball)
	Garlic	To taste
	EVOO	2 tablespoons (1 shot glass)
Day 3	Alaskan halibut	3–4 ounces (1 deck of cards)
	Quinoa	½ cup (½ baseball)
	Garlic	To taste
	EVOO	2 tablespoons (1 shot glass)
Day 4	Skinless turkey breast	3–4 ounces (1 deck of cards)
	Barley	½ cup (½ baseball)
	Onion	¼ medium (½ baseball)
	EVOO	2 tablespoons (1 shot glass)
Day 5	Brown rice	½ cup (½ baseball)
	Leeks	½ cup (½ baseball)
	Yellow corn	½ cup (½ baseball)
	EVOO	2 tablespoons (1 shot glass)
Day 6	Canned chunk light tuna	3–4 ounces (1 deck of cards)
	Whole grain bread	2 slices
	Scallions	½ cup (½ baseball)
	EVOO	2 tablespoons (1 shot glass)
Day 7	Skinless turkey breast	3–4 ounces (1 deck of cards)
	Wild rice	½ cup (½ baseball)
	Garlic	To taste
	EVOO	2 tablespoons (1 shot glass)

Week 4: Control Inflammation Daily Exercise Planner

	Exercise	Set Reminders
Day 1	Walk	20 minutes
	Power Stairs	7 minutes
	Heel to Fanny	3 sets of 15
	Isometric Curl	15 times with both arms
	Isometric Extension	15 times with both arms
	Ball Squeeze	20 times
	Steering Wheel Squeeze	10 times
Day 2	Walk	20 minutes
	Heel to Fanny	3 sets of 15
	Sit-up/Crunch	3 sets of 20
	Isometric Curl	15 times with both arms
	Isometric Extension	15 times with both arms
	Bicep Curl	3 sets of 10
	Tricep Extension	3 sets of 10
Day 3	Walk	20 minutes
	Power Stairs	7 minutes
	Ball Squeeze	20 times
	Stand Up/Sit Down/Wall Sit	3 sets of 15
	Steering Wheel Squeeze	10 times
Day 4	Walk	20 minutes
	Heel to Fanny	3 sets of 15
	Sit-up/Crunch	3 sets of 20
	Isometric Curl	15 times with both arms
	Isometric Extension	15 times with both arms
	Ball Squeeze	20 times per day
	Stand Up/Sit Down/Wall Sit	3 sets of 15
Day 5	Walk	20 minutes
	Power Stairs	7 minutes
	Isometric Curl	15 times with both arms
	Isometric Extension	15 times with both arms
	Ball Squeeze	20 times
	Bicep Curl	3 sets of 10
	Tricep Extension	3 sets of 10

(continued)

	Exercise	Set Reminders
Day 6	Walk	20 minutes
	Heel to Fanny	3 sets of 15
	Sit-up/Crunch	3 sets of 20
	Ball Squeeze	20 times
	Stand Up/Sit Down/Wall Sit	3 sets of 15
	Steering Wheel Squeeze	10 times
Day 7	Walk	20 minutes
	Power Stairs	7 minutes
	Isometric Curl	15 times with both arms
	Isometric Extension	15 times with both arms
	Bicep Curl	3 sets of 10
	Tricep Extension	3 sets of 10

Week 4: Control Inflammation Shopping List

*(Always look for no-salt-added or
low-sodium products.)*

Wild salmon + Sidekicks
Skinless turkey breast + Sidekick
Fresh garlic, onions + Sidekicks

Canned Albacore Tuna
- Bumble Bee Solid White Albacore Tuna in Water
- Chicken of the Sea Chunk Light Tuna in Canola Oil
- Chicken of the Sea Low-Sodium Chunk White Albacore Tuna
- Kirkland Solid White Albacore Tuna Packed in Water
- StarKist Solid White Albacore Tuna in Water
- Trader Joe's White Solid Albacore Tuna (reduced sodium)

Canned Clams and Crab
- Sea Watch Chopped Sea Clams
- Trader Joe's Chopped Sea Clams
- Trader Joe's Crab Meat

Canned Salmon

- Bumble Bee Alaskan Pink Salmon
- Bumble Bee Alaskan Sockeye Red Salmon
- Chicken of the Sea Pink Salmon
- Crown Prince Fancy Alaskan Pink Salmon (low sodium) www.crownprince.com
- Libby's Red Salmon
- Trader Joe's Alaskan Pink Salmon
- Trader Joe's Red Salmon
- Vital Choice Wild Red Sockeye Salmon (no sodium added)

Cold Cereal

- Alpen Naturally Delicious Swiss Style Cereal (low fat)
- Alpen Swiss Style Cereal (no added sugar or salt)
- Arrowhead Mills Organic Spelt Flakes
- Back to Nature Granola www.organicmilling.com
- Back to Nature Ultra Flax
- Barbara's Bite Size Shredded Oats Crunchy Wholegrain Cereal www.barbarasbakery.com
- Barbara's Grain Shop High Fiber Cereal
- Bob's Red Mill Whole Ground Flaxseed Meal
- Bob's Red Mill Natural Raw Wheat Germ
- Breadshop's Cranberry Crunch Muesli
- Breadshop's Granola Crunchy Oat Bran with Almonds and Raisins
- Cheerios
- Familia Low-Fat Granola
- Familia No Added Sugar Swiss Muesli
- Familia Original Recipe Muesli
- Galaxy Granola Radically Raspberry www.galaxygranola.com
- Health Valley Organic Amaranth Flakes
- Health Valley Organic Multigrain Flakes
- Health Valley Organic Oat Bran Flakes
- Health Valley Organic Oat Bran O's
- Kashi Go Lean Good Friends Cereal
- Kashi Go Lean Protein and High Fiber Cereal

- Kashi Go Lean Seven Whole Grains and Sesame
- Kellogg's Complete Oat Bran Flakes
- Kellogg's Complete Wheat Bran Flakes
- Kretschmer Toasted Wheat Germ
- Nature's Path Heritage O's
- Nature's Path Organic Blueberry Muesli
- Nature's Path Organic Optimum Power Breakfast Cereal—Flax-Soy-Blueberry
- Organic Fiber 7 Multigrain Flakes
- Post Grape-Nuts Flakes
- Post Shredded Wheat 'N Bran
- Trader Joe's Organic Golden Flax Cereal
- Uncle Sam Cereal—Toasted Whole Grain Wheat Flakes with Crispy Whole Flaxseed
- Weetabix Organic Cereal

Cooked Cereal

- Bob's Red Mill 7 Grain Hot Cereal www.bobsredmill.com
- Hodgson Mill All Natural Oat Bran Hot Cereal
- McCann's Imported Quick Cooking Irish Oatmeal
- McCann's Instant Irish Oatmeal (regular flavor)
- McCann's Steel Cut Irish Oatmeal
- Mother's 100% Natural Rolled Oats
- Mother's 100% Natural Whole-Grain Barley
- Quaker Instant Oatmeal (original)
- Quaker Oat Bran Hot Cereal
- Quaker Old-Fashioned Oats
- Quaker Quick Oats
- Silver Palate Thick and Rough Oatmeal
- Stone-Buhr 7 Grain Cereal www.s-bcereals.com
- Stone-Buhr 7 Grain Cereal Mates
- Wheatena Toasted Wheat Cereal

Extra Virgin Olive Oil

- Eliki Organic Extra Virgin Olive Oil www.elikioliveoil.com
- Sonoma Farm Organic Garlic Infused Extra Virgin Olive Oil www.sonomafarm.com
- Spectrum Extra Virgin Olive Oil (first cold press) www.spectrumorganics. com

Frozen Fish

- High Liner Atlantic Cod Fillets
- Kauai Shrimp Fresh Island Fish www.freshislandfish.com
- Ocean Beauty Wild Alaskan Salmon
- Omstead Fresh Water Cleaned Smelt 519-825-7144
- Vital Choice Alaskan Fish Fillets (multiple varieties)
- Whole Foods Market wild sockeye salmon, scallops, shrimp, yellowfin tuna steaks, wild Alaskan cod fillets

Ground Flaxseed/Wheat Germ

- Bob's Red Mill Whole Ground Flaxseed
- Kretschmer Original Toasted Wheat Germ

Sardines

- Beach Cliff Sardines in Soybean Oil
- Bela Olhão Portugal Lightly Smoked Sardines in Olive Oil
- Crown Prince One Layer Brisling Sardines in Oil
- Crown Prince Skinless and Boneless Sardines in Olive Oil
- King Oscar Extra Small Sardines in Purest Virgin Olive Oil
- Yankee Clipper Lightly Smoked Sardines in Lemon Sauce
- Yankee Clipper Lightly Smoked Sardines in Tomato Sauce

Whole Grains

- Fantastic Organic Whole Wheat Couscous www.fantasticfoods.com
- Lundberg Family Farms Organic Long Grain Brown Rice www.lundberg.com
- Lundberg Family Farms Organic Short Grain Brown Rice
- Lundberg Family Farms Organic Wild Rice Blend
- Ralph's Whole Wheat Whole Grain Rotini
- Ronzoni Healthy Harvest 7 Grain Pasta
- Ronzoni Healthy Harvest Whole Wheat Blend Pasta
- Texmati Long Grain American Basmati Brown Rice
- Trader Joe's Basmati Rice Medley
- Trader Joe's Brown Rice Medley
- Trader Joe's California Brown Aromatic Rice
- Trader Joe's Red Rice
- Trader Joe's Rice Trilogy

Week 5: Keep Up Appearances Daily Food Planner

	Food Suggestion	Daily Servings
Day 1	Dark chocolate	100 calories
	Avocado	⅓ avocado
	Orange	1 medium (1 baseball)
	Raisins	2 heaping tablespoons (1 heaping shot glass)
	Tomato	1 medium (1 baseball)
	Pumpkin	½ cup (½ baseball)
	Tea	4 cups
	Vitamin C	250–550 mg up to 4 times a day
	Vitamin E	100–200 IU a day
	Vitamin A	Maximum of 3000 IU a day
Day 2	Asparagus	½ cup (½ baseball)
	Pink grapefruit	1 medium (1 baseball)
	Tomato paste	2 tablespoons (1 shot glass)
	Carrots	½ cup (½ baseball)
	Tea	4 cups

	Food Suggestion	**Daily Servings**
	Vitamin C	250–550 mg up to 4 times a day
	Vitamin E	100–200 IU a day
	Vitamin A	Maximum of 3000 IU a day
Day 3	Dark chocolate	100 calories
	EVOO	2 tablespoons (1 shot glass)
	Blueberries	1 cup (1 baseball)
	Tomato	1 medium (1 baseball)
	Orange bell pepper	½ cup (½ baseball)
	Tea	4 cups
	Vitamin C	250–550 mg up to 4 times a day
	Vitamin E	100–200 IU a day
	Vitamin A	Maximum of 3000 IU a day
Day 4	Dark chocolate	100 calories
	Artichoke	½ cup (½ baseball)
	Kumquats	2 small kumquats
	Tomato paste	2 tablespoons (1 shot glass)
	Butternut squash	½ cup (½ baseball)
	Tea	4 cups
	Vitamin C	250–550 mg up to 4 times a day
	Vitamin E	100–200 IU a day
	Vitamin A	Maximum of 3000 IU a day
Day 5	Avocado	⅓ avocado
	Orange juice	½ cup (4 ounces)
	Dried cranberries	2 heaping tablespoons (1 heaping shot glass)
	Sweet potato	½ cup (½ baseball)
	Tea	4 cups
	Vitamin C	250–550 mg up to 4 times a day
	Vitamin E	100–200 IU a day
	Vitamin A	Maximum of 3000 IU a day
Day 6	Dark chocolate	100 calories
	Lemon juice	½ cup (4 ounces)
	Currants	2 heaping tablespoons (1 heaping shot glass)

(continued)

	Food Suggestion	**Daily Servings**
Day 6 (*cont.*)	Tomato	1 medium (1 baseball)
	Pumpkin	½ cup (½ baseball)
	Tea	4 cups
	Vitamin C	250–550 mg up to 4 time a day
	Vitamin E	100–200 IU a day
	Vitamin A	Maximum of 3000 IU a day
Day 7	Dark chocolate	100 calories
	EVOO	2 tablespoons (1 shot glass)
	Orange	1 medium (1 baseball)
	Persimmon	1 medium (1 baseball)
	Carrots	½ cup (½ baseball)
	Tea	4 cups
	Vitamin C	250–550 mg up to 4 times a day
	Vitamin E	100–200 IU a day
	Vitamin A	Maximum of 3000 IU a day

Week 5: Keep Up Appearances Daily Exercise Planner

	Exercise	**Set Reminders**
Day 1	Walk	25 minutes
	Power Stairs	10 minutes
	Heel to Fanny	3 sets of 20
	Isometric Curl	20 times with both arms; hold for 20 seconds
	Isometric Extension	20 times with both arms; hold for 20 seconds
	Ball Squeeze	20 times a day
	Steering Wheel Squeeze	3 sets of 15
	Waist Twist	3 sets of 20
	Side Bends	3 sets of 20
	Platysma Rock	10 times
Day 2	Walk	25 minutes
	Heel to Fanny	3 sets of 20
	Sit-up/Crunch	3 sets of 30
	Isometric Curl	20 times with both arms; hold for 20 seconds

	Exercise	Set Reminders
	Isometric Extension	20 times with both arms; hold for 20 seconds
	Bicep Curl	3 sets of 10; add weight
	Tricep Extension	3 sets of 10; add weight
	Bicycle	30 seconds
Day 3	Walk	25 minutes
	Power Stairs	10 minutes
	Ball Squeeze	20 times
	Stand Up/Sit Down/Wall Sit	Unlimited times
	Steering Wheel Squeeze	3 sets of 15
	Waist Twist	3 sets of 20
	Side Bends	3 sets of 20
	Platysma Rock	10 times
Day 4	Walk	25 minutes
	Heel to Fanny	3 sets of 20
	Sit-up/Crunch	3 sets of 30
	Isometric Curl	20 times with both arms; hold for 20 seconds
	Isometric Extension	20 times with both arms; hold for 20 seconds
	Ball Squeeze	20 times
	Stand Up/Sit Down/Wall Sit	Unlimited times
	Bicycle	30 seconds
Day 5	Walk	25 minutes
	Power Stairs	10 minutes
	Isometric Curl	20 times with both arms; hold for 20 seconds
	Isometric Extension	20 times with both arms; hold for 20 seconds
	Ball Squeeze	20 times
	Bicep Curl	3 sets of 10; add weight
	Tricep Extension	3 sets of 10; add weight
	Waist Twist	3 sets of 20
	Side Bends	3 sets of 20
	Platysma Rock	10 times
Day 6	Walk	25 minutes
	Heel to Fanny	3 sets of 20
	Sit-Up/Crunch	3 sets of 30

(continued)

	Exercise	**Set Reminders**
Day 6	Ball Squeeze	20 times
(cont.)	Stand Up/Sit Down/Wall Sit	Unlimited times
	Steering Wheel Squeeze	3 sets of 15
	Bicycle	30 seconds
Day 7	Walk	25 minutes
	Power Stairs	10 minutes
	Isometric Curl	20 times with both arms; hold for 20 seconds
	Isometric Extension	20 times with both arms; hold for 20 seconds
	Bicep Curl	3 sets of 10; add weight
	Tricep Extension	3 sets of 10; add weight
	Waist Twist	3 sets of 20
	Side Bends	3 sets of 20
	Platysma Rock	10 times

Week 5: Keep Up Appearances Shopping List

*(Always look for no-salt-added or
low-sodium products.)*

Fresh tomatoes + Sidekicks
Fresh oranges + Sidekicks
Fresh avocados + Sidekicks
Fresh pumpkin + Sidekicks

Black Tea
- Bigelow Tea
- Celestial Seasonings Tea
- Choice Organic Tea
- Lipton Tea
- Numi Organic Tea
- Stash Tea
- Tazo Tea
- Twinings Tea
- Yogi Tea

Canned Pumpkin
- Libby's 100% Pure Pumpkin

Canned Tomato Products

- Classico Di Napoli Spicy Red Pepper Pasta Sauce
- Classico DiNapoli Tomato and Basil Pasta Sauce
- Colavita 100% Natural Marinara Sauce www.colavita.com
- Del Monte Diced Tomatoes (no salt added)
- Emeril's Roasted Red Pepper Pasta Sauce
- Hunt's Tomato Sauce (no salt added)
- Muir Glen Organic Chunky Tomato and Herb Pasta Sauce
- Muir Glen Organic Chunky Tomato Sauce www.muirglen.com
- Muir Glen Organic Crushed Tomatoes with Basil
- Muir Glen Organic Ground Peeled Tomatoes
- Muir Glenn Organic Tomato Paste
- Muir Glen Organic Tomato Puree
- Muir Glen Organic Whole Peeled Tomatoes
- Private Selection (PS) Organic Tomato Paste (Kroger's)
- Ralph's Peeled Tomatoes (diced, no salt added)
- Ralph's Peeled Tomatoes (whole, no salt added)
- Ralph's Tomato Sauce (no salt added)
- S&W Petite-Cut Diced Tomatoes in Rich, Thick Juice
- S&W Ready-Cut Tomatoes (diced, no salt added)
- Walnut Acres Organic Zesty Basil Pasta Sauce www.walnutacres.com

Dark Chocolate

- Cadbury Royal Dark Chocolate
- Dagoba Organic Cacao Powder www.dagobachocolate .com
- Dina's Dark Chocolate with Green Tea www.dinakhadev.com
- Dove Silky Dark Chocolate
- Endangered Species Chocolate Company Wolf Bar (with cranberries and almonds)
- Hershey's Special Dark Chocolate

- Newman's Own Sweet Dark Chocolate
- Rapunzel Organic Chocolate Powder www.rapunzel.com

- SuperFoodsRx Premium Dark Chocolate www.superfoodsrx.com

Dried Fruit

- Elizabeth's Natural Cranberries 631-243-1626
- Maiani Kirkland Pitted Dried Plums (Costco)
- Melissa's Organic Dried Bing Cherries www.melissas.com
- Melissa's Organic Dried Cranberries
- Ocean Spray Craisins Original Sweetened Dried Cranberries
- Sun-Maid Raisins
- Sunsweet Pitted Dates
- Sunsweet Premium Prunes
- Sunview Red Seedless Raisins

www.sunviewmarketing.com
- Trader Joe's Berry Medley
- Trader Joe's Bing Cherries
- Trader Joe's California Organic Thompson Seedless Raisins
- Trader Joe's Dried Blueberries
- Trader Joe's Extra Large High Moisture Prunes
- Trader Joe's Non-Sorbate Pitted Prunes
- Trader Joe's Organic Imported Apricots

Extra Virgin Olive Oil

- Eliki Organic Extra Virgin Olive Oil www.elikioil.com
- Sonoma Farm Organic Garlic Infused Extra Virgin Olive Oil

www.sonomafarm.com
- Spectrum Extra Virgin Olive Oil (first cold press) www.spectrumorganics.com

Green Tea

- Bigelow Green Tea: plain, peach, mint, lemon, variety pack

- Celestial Seasonings Green: Authentic, Honey Lemon Ginseng

- Choice Organic Tea
- Good Earth Green Tea Blend with Lemongrass
- Lipton Green Tea
- Mighty Leaf Organic Green Teas: Tropical Green, Hoijicha
- Numi Organic Green Tea
- Salada 100% Green Tea
- Stash Chai Green Tea
- Tazo China Green Tips, Zen
- Twinings Green
- Yogi Green Tea

Week 6: Preserve Your Senses Daily Food Planner

	Food Suggestion	Daily Servings
Day 1	Pomegranate	½ cup (4 ounces) 100% juice
	Blueberries	1 cup (1 baseball)
	Walnuts	1 handful (1 layer on your palm)
	Spinach	2 cups raw (2 baseballs)
	Orange	1 medium (1 baseball)
	Wheat germ	2 tablespoons (1 shot glass)
Day 2	Strawberries	2 cups (2 baseballs)
	Almonds	1 handful (1 layer on your palm)
	Romaine lettuce	2 cups (2 baseballs)
	Kiwi	1 kiwi
	Orange juice	½ cup (4 ounces)
	Wheat germ	2 tablespoons (1 shot glass)
Day 3	Pomegranate	½ cup (4 ounces) 100% juice
	Cherries	1 cup (1 baseball)
	Pistachios	½ handful (1 layer on half of your palm)
	Kale	1 cup steamed (1 baseball)
	Pink grapefruit	½ grapefruit
	Wheat germ	2 tablespoons (1 shot glass)
	Almonds	½ handful (1 layer on half of your palm)
Day 4	Pomegranate	½ cup (4 ounces) 100% juice
		(continued)

	Food Suggestion	**Daily Servings**
Day 4 (*cont.*)	Purple grapes	1 cup (1 baseball)
	Pumpkin seeds	1 handful (1 layer on your palm)
	Arugula	2 cups raw (2 baseballs)
	Kiwi	1 kiwi
	Lemon	½ cup lemon juice
Day 5	Blueberries	1 cup (1 baseball)
	Cashews	½ handful (1 layer on half of your palm)
	Turnip greens	1 cup steamed (1 baseball)
	Tangerine	2 tangerines
	Wheat germ	2 tablespoons (1 shot glass)
	Almonds	1 handful (1 layer on ½ your palm)
Day 6	Pomegranate	½ cup (4 ounces) 100% juice
	Cran-raspberry juice	1 cup (8 ounces)
	Pecans	1 handful (1 layer on your palm)
	Spinach	2 cups raw (2 baseballs)
	Kiwi	1 kiwi
	Pink grapefruit	½ grapefruit
Day 7	Pomegranate	½ cup (4 ounces) 100% juice
	Açai-berry/blueberry juice	½ cup (4 ounces)
	Peanuts	½ handful (1 layer on half of your palm)
	Orange	1 medium (1 baseball)
	Wheat germ	2 tablespoons (1 shot glass)
	Almonds	½ handful (1 layer on half of your palm)
	Spinach	2 cups raw (2 baseballs)

Week 6: Preserve Your Senses Daily Exercise Planner

	Exercise	**Set Reminders**
Day 1	Walk	30 minutes
	Power Stairs	15 minutes; increase speed
	Heel to Fanny	3 sets of 20; add weight

	Exercise	Set Reminders
	Isometric Curl	25 times with both arms; hold for 20 seconds
	Isometric Extension	25 times with both arms; hold for 20 seconds
	Ball Squeeze	20 times
	Steering Wheel Squeeze	3 sets of 20
	Waist Twist	3 sets of 30–50
	Side Bends	3 sets of 30–50
	Platysma Rock	20 times
	Push-ups	3 sets of 5
	Pull-ups	10 in a row
Day 2	Walk	30 minutes
	Heel to Fanny	3 sets of 20; add weight
	Sit-up/Crunch	5 sets of 30
	Isometric Curl	25 times with both arms; hold for 20 seconds
	Isometric Extension	25 times with both arms; hold for 20 seconds
	Bicep Curl	3 sets of 10; add weight
	Tricep Extension	3 sets of 10; add weight
	Bicycle	60 seconds
Day 3	Walk	30 minutes
	Power Stairs	15 minutes; increase speed
	Ball Squeeze	20 times
	Stand Up/Sit Down/Wall Sit	Unlimited times
	Steering Wheel Squeeze	3 sets of 20
	Waist Twist	3 sets of 30–50
	Side Bends	3 sets of 30–50
	Platysma Rock	20 times
	Push-ups	3 sets of 5
	Pull-ups	10 in a row
Day 4	Walk	30 minutes
	Heel to Fanny	3 sets of 20; add weight
	Sit-up/Crunch	5 sets of 30
	Isometric Curl	25 times with both arms; hold for 20 seconds
	Isometric Extension	25 times with both arms; hold for 20 seconds

(continued)

	Exercise	**Set Reminders**
Day 4 (*cont.*)	Ball Squeeze	20 times
	Stand Up/Sit Down/Wall Sit	Unlimited times
	Bicycle	30 seconds
Day 5	Walk	30 minutes
	Power Stairs	15 minutes; increase speed
	Isometric Curl	25 times with both arms; hold for 20 seconds
	Isometric Extension	25 times with both arms; hold for 20 seconds
	Ball Squeeze	20 times
	Bicep Curl	3 sets of 10; add weight
	Tricep Extension	3 sets of 10; add weight
	Waist Twist	3 sets of 30–50
	Side Bends	3 sets of 30–50
	Platysma Rock	20 times
Day 6	Walk	30 minutes
	Heel to Fanny	3 sets of 20; add weight
	Sit-up/Crunch	5 sets of 30
	Ball Squeeze	20 times
	Stand Up/Sit Down/Wall Sit	Unlimited times
	Steering Wheel Squeeze	3 sets of 20
	Bicycle	60 seconds
	Push-ups	3 sets of 5
	Pull-ups	10 in a row
Day 7	Walk	30 minutes
	Power Stairs	15 minutes; increase speed
	Isometric Curl	25 times with both arms; hold for 20 seconds
	Isometric Extension	25 times with both arms; hold for 20 seconds
	Bicep Curl	3 sets of 10; add weight
	Tricep Extension	3 sets of 10; add weight
	Waist Twist	3 sets of 30–50
	Side Bends	3 sets of 30–50
	Platysma Rock	20 times

Week 6: Preserve Your Senses Shopping List

*(Always look for no-salt-added or
low-sodium products.)*

Fresh blueberries + Sidekicks
Fresh spinach + Sidekicks
Fresh kiwis
Fresh oranges + Sidekicks

Bottled Juice

- Columbia Gorge Certified Organic Juices (multiple flavors) www.CoGoJuice.com
- Kedem Concord 100% Pure Grape Juice
- Kirkland Cranberry-Grape 100% Juice Blend
- Kirkland 100% Grape Juice
- Minute Maid 100% Pure Grape Juice
- Mountain Sun Pure Cranberry Juice (100% pure unsweetened cranberry juice is tart, so mix it with another, sweeter 100% pure fruit juice)
- Ocean Spray Premium 100% Cranberry Juice
- R.W. Knudsen Family Just Concord
- R.W. Knudsen Family Organic Cranberry Juice
- Trader Joe's All Natural Triple Berry Juice 100% Juice Blend from Pomegranates, Blueberries, and Cranberries
- Trader Joe's 100% Unfiltered Concord Grape Juice
- Walnut Acres Certified Organic Concord Grape Juice
- Walnut Acres Certified Organic Wild Cranberry Juice
- Welch's 100% Grape Juice

Frozen Fruits and Vegetables

- Cascadian Farm Organic Blackberries www.cascadianfarm.com
- Cascadian Farm Organic Chinese-Style Stir Fry
- Cascadian Farm Organic Garden Blend Premium Vegetables
- Cascadian Farm Organic Harvest Berries

- Cascadian Farm Organic Red Raspberries
- Cascadian Farm Organic Strawberries
- Flav•R•Pac Deluxe Berry Mix www.norpac.com
- NutriVerde California Blend (broccoli and cauliflower florets with carrots) www.nutriverde.com
- Trader Joe's frozen fruits and frozen vegetables (multiple varieties)
- Whole Foods brand frozen fruits and vegetables

Nuts and Seeds

- Ann's House of Nuts Unsalted Dry-Roasted Peanuts
- Elizabeth's Natural No-Salt Roasted in Shell Pumpkin Seeds
- Elizabeth's Natural Pecans
- Elizabeth's Natural Raw Almonds
- Elizabeth's Natural Raw Cashews
- Elizabeth's Natural Raw Hulled Sunflower Seeds
- Elizabeth's Natural Walnuts
- Hoody's Classic Roast Peanuts (Original Nut House Brand)
- Kirkland Almonds
- Kirkland Pecan Halves
- Kirkland Walnuts
- Old Tyme Peanuts (no salt or oil)
- Planters Unsalted Peanuts
- Trader Joe's California Premium Walnut Halves
- Trader Joe's California Walnut Halves and Pieces
- Trader Joe's Dry Roasted and Unsalted Pistachios
- Trader Joe's Raw Pecan Pieces
- Trader Joe's Raw Sunflower Seeds
- Trader Joe's Roasted and Unsalted Whole Cashews

Wheat Germ

- Kretschmer Original Toasted Wheat Germ

14

Preventing the 6 Major Causes of Death

TOP 22 TIPS FOR PREVENTING (OR LIVING WITH) CARDIOVASCULAR DISEASE (HEART ATTACK AND STROKE)
THE SUPERHEALTH WAY

Tip #1: No cigarettes or exposure to secondhand smoke.

Tip #2: Become an environmentalist (see Chapter 4).

Tip #3: Get seven to eight hours of sleep a night (see Chapter 6).

Tip #4: Watch your weight and waistline (see Chapter 5). Abdominal obesity is a significant risk factor for atherosclerosis and a significant warning for future heart disease. Abdominal obesity is associated with early atherosclerosis as measured by the coronary calcium score in African American and white young adults. Coronary artery calcification is a risk marker for atherosclerosis, coronary heart disease, and cardiovascular events.

Tip #5: Burn those calories. Get in forty-five to ninety minutes of physical activity most days, including resistance exercise two to three times weekly.

Tip #6: DASH your way to lower blood pressure. The Dietary Approaches to Stop Hypertension (DASH) diet (fruits, vegetables, whole grains, nuts and seeds, low-fat and nonfat dairy high in dietary calcium and magnesium) has been shown to effectively lower blood pressure and cardiovascular risk factors. This diet is full of SuperFoods and is also similar to the classic Mediterranean diet. When combined with sodium restriction (1500 milligrams) this type of dietary pattern can lower systolic blood pressure by as much as 10 to 12 mmHg! See www.nhlbi.nih.gov/health/public/heart/hbp/dash.

Tip #7: Eat your vegetables (and fruits). There are many studies reporting a significant decreased risk for stroke, hypertension, and heart attack in people who consistently consume their fruits and vegetables.

Tip #8: Be a carotenoid king or queen. Alphacarotene and beta-carotene are two best bets for decreasing your risk of cardiovascular disease (by about 20 percent), so pumpkin, carrots, butternut squash, and sweet potatoes need to make regular appearances on your plate. And don't forget the other carotenoids, such as lycopene, lutein, and zeaxanthin, as some studies also suggest that it is the overall carotenoid blood level that is the key. Carotenoids also possess anti-inflammatory properties and help keep the endothelial cells (cells lining the blood vessels) at optimum function. See the SuperNutrients and SuperFoods list (page 244) for daily goals to help achieve the most protective amounts.

Tip #9: Take an antioxidant "bath" with every meal. At the end of the day there is nothing like a nice warm bath to make you feel better. At the end of a meal there is nothing like a "bath" of antioxidants to keep you feeling your best. There is increasing evidence that postprandial (after eating) fats in the blood and the oxidative stress that often occurs after a non-SuperFoods meal are a more important measure of what's doing you harm than your normal cholesterol screening. Therefore, the food in every meal should be accompanied by foods and/or liquids (preferably both) that increase antioxidant capacity in your blood. Picture all the food you eat taking a bath in an antioxidant "broth" of blueberries (and all those sidekicks), kiwis, grapes, cherries, pomegranates, and their juices (100 percent, of course), and that should help you accomplish this goal. Foods that decrease oxidative stress in humans include blueberries, kiwis, grape juice, red wine, tomatoes, tomato juice, tomato sauce, polyphenol-rich fruit juices, spinach, Brussels sprouts, garlic, green tea, extra virgin olive oil, soymilk, quercetin-rich foods (see page 335), cruciferous vegetables, and sprouts, and consuming at least twelve servings of fruits and vegetables a day.

In a study involving middle-aged people with at least one documented risk factor for cardiovascular disease, subjects were given 100 grams of berries (1 cup of blueberries = 140 grams) plus one small glass of 100 percent berry drink with lunch and dinner every day for two months. The berries included bilberries (European blueberries), chokecherries, red raspberries, black currants, strawberries, and lingonberries (similar to cranberries). The results were favorable changes in platelet function, HDL cholesterol, and blood pressure. The authors of the study concluded that "regular consumption of berries may play a role in the prevention of cardiovascular disease."

Tip #10: Raise your intake of potassium; lower your intake of sodium. See the table for high-potassium foods (page 275) and my favorite store-bought low-sodium foods (page 268).

Tip #11: Love those nuts and seeds. Especially walnuts (plus almonds, pistachios, sesame seeds, peanuts, pumpkin and sunflower seeds, macadamia nuts, pecans, hazelnuts, and cashews). Aim for 1 to 1½ ounces, five times a week. Make sure the nuts have no added salt or oil.

Tip #12: Love those healthy fats. Bring on the nuts and seeds, avocados, wild salmon, sardines, tuna, first-cold-pressed extra virgin olive oil, canola oil, whole grains, dark chocolate, and small amounts of corn oil, soybean oil, and high oleic (monounsaturated) sunflower and safflower oil. Portion control is in, and avoidance is out. A study using snack chips cooked in corn oil (a polyunsaturated fat, low in saturated fatty acids and containing no trans fatty acids) led to improvements in lipid profiles that are associated with reductions in cardiovascular disease risk.

Tip #13: Eat like an Alaskan brown bear. Favor blueberries (plus sidekicks, purple grapes, cranberries, boysenberries, raspberries, strawberries, fresh currants, blackberries, cherries, and all other varieties of fresh, frozen, or freeze-dried berries) and wild salmon (plus sidekicks, Alaskan halibut, canned chunk light or albacore tuna, sardines, herring, farmed trout, sea bass, oysters, and clams [farmed or wild]). Aim for one to two cups of berries most days and 3 to 4 ounces of fish, two to four times a week.

Tip #14: Drink tea. Aim for a minimum of four cups a day of white, green, black, oolong, or rooibos (a naturally decaffeinated South African tea with high levels of antioxidants).

Tip #15: "Thin" your blood naturally. To do so, favor kiwis, red wine, soybeans, cayenne pepper, garlic, berry mixtures (including blueberries and sidekicks), sea vegetables (such as kelp), tomato products, and omega-3 fatty acids. The effect of kiwis and tomato products lasts only about four hours, but a consistent daily intake of fruits and vegetables will raise the blood level of salicylates (an anti-inflammatory/anti-platelet) found naturally in these foods.

Tip #16: Bring on the "B"s plus choline and betaine. Although several recent trials concluded that vitamin therapy designed to lower homocysteine levels is not effective in reducing the risk of cardiovascular events, further analysis of this relationship suggests that a final verdict has not yet been reached. Taking a multivitamin that contains vitamins B_6 and B_{12}, and folic acid, as well as consuming foods containing the "new nutrients on the block," betaine and choline, may be beneficial. Betaine is found in spinach and whole grain bran, while choline is found in eggs, poultry, fish, broccoli, soy, cauliflower, low-fat milk, potatoes, green beans, legumes, cashews, peanuts, almonds, yogurt, cod, shrimp, salmon, spinach, whole grains, and avocados (see page 272 for a more complete list). It's also found in beef and pork, but I recommend you limit your intake of red meat (preferably grass-fed or buffalo) to a maximum of four ounces or less a week. While dietary choline and betaine have been studied for years, a new study reports higher dietary intake of these nutrients reduces inflammatory biomarkers including our old friends C-reactive protein and IL-6, and is also associated with a decrease in plasma homocysteine, atherosclerosis, colorectal adenoma (benign tumor), and breast cancer. For those sixty-five and over I recommend achieving a total supplement goal of 300 micrograms a day of vitamin B_{12}.

Tip #17: Consume 10 to 15 grams of whole food soy protein. Include soybeans, edamame, soy nuts, soymilk, miso, tofu, or soy flour most days.

Tip #18: Love those whole grains. Habitual whole grain consumption has been shown to lower the risk for diabetes, obesity, metabolic syndrome, various cancers, endothelial dysfunction, oxidative stress and related inflammatory markers, and cardiovascular disease. A recent study has shown that whole grain intake is inversely associated with carotid artery wall thickness (a noninvasive marker of bodywide atherosclerosis). And in another study of 28,926 female health professionals age forty-five or older, those who consumed four or more servings of whole grains a day (as opposed to those consuming less than .5 servings a day) had a 23 percent decreased risk of developing high blood pressure. Regular intake of whole grains produces a 20 to 40 percent reduction in the risk of coronary heart disease and a 20 to 30 percent reduction in the risk for diabetes. Aim for a minimum 10 grams of whole grain fiber most days and 3 to 4 grams of whole grain bran most days (see the whole grain fiber list on page 91 and Super-Foods list for Oats plus Sidekicks on page 249). In the United States, the current intake of whole grains is less than one serving a day, with five servings of refined grains a day. There's also a recent study showing an inverse relationship between whole grain intake and deaths related to inflammatory diseases such as nonmalignant respiratory disease, infectious disease, rheumatoid arthritis, chronic obstructive pulmonary disease, asthma, ulcerative colitis, and Crohn's disease. People who had the highest whole grain intake had a 35 percent reduction of death from those diseases.

Tip #19: Control your blood sugar. A tight control of blood sugar is mandatory for achieving and sustaining SuperHealth and for avoiding most of the chronic diseases plaguing us at present. Oats and barley are especially good (along with other whole grains) for regulating postprandial blood sugar, not only with the meal in which they are consumed but also with subsequent meals during the course of the day and overnight when consumed in the evening.

Tip #20: Add 2 to 4 tablespoons per day of whole ground flaxseed meal to your meals. This is the easiest way to get whole food alpha-linolenic acid (ALA), the plant source of long-chain omega-3 fatty acids. For maximum prevention of cardiovascular disease, or for those suffering from this condition, it is very important to consume adequate daily amounts of both alpha-linolenic acid and fish oil with its EPA/DHA. Flaxseed contains the highest amounts of ALA in the plant kingdom, followed by walnuts. Add flaxseed meal into hot or dry cereal, applesauce (no sugar added), or R.W. Knudsen's Very Veggie Vegetable Cocktail Juice (low sodium). Green leafy vegetables like spinach and purslane are good dietary sources of this important fatty acid.

Tip #21: Supplement your health. For best protection, you should be consuming 500 to 1000 milligrams a day for women and 1000 to 2000 milligrams a day for men of EPA/DHA (fish oil). Ideally this quantity is reached through a combination of wild Alaskan salmon plus sidekicks and fish oil supplements (see www.superfoodsrx.com or www.maxivision.com for information about state-of-the-art multivitamin, mineral, and antioxidant supplements).

Tip #22: Indulge in dark chocolate. This SuperFood is super-good for the cardiovascular system. Dark chocolate causes a vasodilation effect (widening of the blood vessels), which leads to statistically significant decreases in systolic and diastolic blood pressure, has a positive effect on reducing platelet reactivity and adhesion tendencies, seems to enhance mood, and can increase coronary artery diameter (thus increasing blood flow). Aim for 40 grams (approximately 1.5 ounces) a day. When buying dark chocolate look for labels stating the cocoa solids content—you want 70 percent or more. You can also buy 100 percent cocoa powder or grind the beans yourself (you can get them from International Harvest, 914-939-5600). Look for nonalkalized cocoa products (alkalization decreases the polyphenol content of the product). For my favorite SuperHealth Hot Chocolate drink, see the recipe on page 280. This may be the tastiest way to lower blood pressure, pick up your mood, and produce an aspirin-like effect on your platelets. No side effect except a decreased risk of cardiovascular disease and all-cause mortality! Here are some great brands of dark chocolate bars:

- Cadbury Royal Dark Chocolate
- Dove Silky Dark Chocolate
- Endangered Species Chocolate Company Wolf Bar (with cranberries and almonds)
- Hershey's Special Dark Mildly Sweet Chocolate
- Newman's Own Organics Sweet Dark Chocolate
- SuperFoodsRx Kitchen 72% Premium Dark Chocolate (nonalkalized and also contains omega-3s) (www.superfoodsrx.com)

TOP 10 TIPS FOR BREAST CANCER PREVENTION

Tip #1: Have a yearly mammogram starting at age forty and a clinical breast exam every year as well. Start breast self-exams at the age of about twenty.

Tip #2: If you're planning on having children, speak with your health-care professional about strategies to keep your weight under control during the pregnancy and to have a normal-weight child at birth. Breast feed for six to twelve months to help ensure a lifetime of SuperHealth for your child and help decrease your risk of breast cancer. Breastfeeding is also a great way to normalize your weight after delivery.

Tip #3: If you have a positive family history of breast cancer, avoid alcohol. If there is no family history and you choose to drink, have a maximum of three drinks a week.

Tip #4: Choose healthy fats (first-cold-pressed extra virgin olive oil, canola oil, fat from nuts and seeds, avocados, and whole grains, wild salmon and sidekicks like Alaskan halibut, canned chunk light or albacore tuna in water, sardines, herring, farmed trout, sea bass, oysters, and clams [farmed or wild]).

Tip #5: Watch your weight and your waist: the mirror tells all. Aim for a stable normal weight during your adult life (see the BMI table on page 340).

Tip #6: Be physically active and burn those calories.

Tip #7: Love those cruciferous veggies (including broccoli, Brussels sprouts, red and green cabbage, kale, turnips, cauliflower, collard greens, bok choy, mustard greens, Swiss chard, rutabaga). Enjoy a wide variety of this class of SuperFoods to achieve the maximum anti–breast cancer effects.

Tip #8: Between your multivitamin, diet, and vitamin D_3 supplements, aim for 1200 to 2000 IU a day of vitamin D, and don't forget to expose your skin (you decide where) to sunlight for ten to twenty minutes at least three to four days a week.

Tip #9: Find a way to enjoy 10 to 15 grams of soy protein (from whole food sources of soy like tofu, soymilk, soy yogurt, soy nuts, edamame, tempeh, and miso) daily (breast cancer survivors should check with their healthcare professionals) and 2 to 4 tablespoons of flaxseed meal most days of the week (especially important for adolescent females). Also enjoy other legumes (such as lentils, chickpeas, black beans, green peas, and pinto beans) several times a week.

Tip #10: Be a fiber-consuming machine: Choose whole fruits and vegetables, whole grain breads and breakfast cereals (look for at least 3 grams of fiber per serving, and be careful of high levels of sugar and salt—see page 264 for fiber sources), brown rice, and legumes (see Tip #9). Avoid refined grains and refined grain products.

TOP 10 TIPS FOR PROSTATE CANCER PREVENTION OR CONTROL

Tip #1: Be physically active in order to control your weight, reduce inflammation, control blood sugar, and reduce serum insulin levels. Exercise is also a great stress reducer: A 2005 study of ninety-three prostate cancer patients found that those who adopted a series of lifestyle changes that included a primarily vegan diet, regular moderate exercise, and yoga and other relaxation techniques scored better on a standard blood test used to monitor prostate cancer growth a year later.

Tip #2: Drink four or more cups of tea a day—white, green, black, oolong, or rooibos. Also drink 4 to 8 ounces of pomegranate juice most days. Studies have shown that this can significantly decrease the growth rate of prostate cancer cells.

Tip #3: Consume 22 milligrams of lycopene from food most if not all days. Keep in mind that the best sources of lycopene are from cooked tomatoes rather than raw. Tomato sauces are the best sources, so the next time you have a slice of pizza (whole grain, of course), ask for a double serving of tomato sauce! (Another tip: Since there appears to be a synergy between tomatoes and broccoli for prostate cancer protection, give yourself an added bang and try having a tomato-broccoli veggie combo.)

Tip #4: Add 2 to 4 tablespoons of ground flaxseed meal to your daily diet (not flaxseed oil). High intakes of alpha-linolenic acid from non–whole food sources and even some food sources may increase the risk of developing prostate cancer, whereas flaxseed meal (a very high source of ALA but also containing all the nutrients of the grain) actually decreases the growth rate of prostate cancer and increases the body's ability to kill already-present prostate cancer cells.

Tip #5: Consume healthy fats and a low intake of saturated fats. Aim for an omega-3 to omega-6 ratio of 1:1 to a maximum of 1:3. Limit saturated fats (check food labels for grams per serving) to less than 7 percent of your total calories a day (that's about 16 grams of saturated fat per 2000 calories). Men with a high percentage of saturated fat in their diet have an increased risk of prostate cancer. Enjoy fat from cold-pressed extra virgin olive oil, canola oil, nuts, seeds, whole grains, and wild salmon.

Tip #6: Love those cruciferous veggies (including broccoli, Brussels sprouts, red and green cabbage, kale, turnips, cauliflower, collard greens, bok choy, mustard greens, Swiss chard, rutabaga).

Tip #7: There is considerable controversy concerning dietary calcium intake from milk products and the risk for prostate cancer. Until this controversy is fully resolved, the best advice is to avoid the possible increased risk of prostate cancer from increased dairy calcium consumption (and perhaps even supplements). Daily adult male dairy guidelines: 1 to 2 cups per day organic nonfat yogurt; 1 cup low-fat or nonfat milk (organic preferred); 1 serving of low-fat cheese no more than three times weekly; 1 serving of low-fat or nonfat cottage cheese no more than three times weekly; 1 container DanActive Immunity. Be sure to consume foods high in dietary vitamin D and reach a total supplementary dose of vitamin D_3 between 1200 and 2000 IU a day. If you supplement with calcium, be sure that your total supplemental dose of calcium a day is less than your total supplemental dose of vitamin D_3 per day. Some studies now say that if you take calcium supplements without vitamin D_3, you may be increasing your risk for prostate cancer.

Tip #8: Consume legumes such as lentils, chickpeas, black beans, green peas, and pinto beans most days, along with 10 to 15 grams of soy protein from whole foods.

Tip #9: Take a well-balanced, up-to-date supplement (see www.superfoodsrx.com, www.maxivision.com) that contains both selenium and vitamin D_3 and all eight types of vitamin E daily. Most vitamin E capsules are made from just one form of the vitamin, but there are actually eight different types of vitamin E, so look for a multivitamin or vitamin E capsule that mentions actual amounts of both tocopherols and tocotrienols. Also consume foods high in vitamin E, including vegetable oils, nuts, green leafy vegetables, wheat germ (see page 258 for additional choices) and fortified cereals.

Tip #10: Have more fun in bed. Some recent studies have shown that men who have ejaculations more than twenty-one times a month (compared to less than seven a month) had a 33 percent lower lifetime risk of prostate cancer.

TOP 10 TIPS FOR COLORECTAL CANCER PREVENTION

Tip #1: Have a colonoscopy—see your health professional for advice on the age at which you should have your first one.

Tip #2: Stay physically active. According to the National Cancer Institute, physical activity most likely influences the development of colon cancer through multiple, perhaps overlapping, biological pathways. Many researchers believe physical activity aids in regular bowel movements, which may decrease the time the colon is exposed to potential carcinogens. Increased physical activity also causes changes in insulin resistance, metabolism, and hormone levels, which may help prevent tumor development.

Tip #3: Limit yourself to a maximum of 3 to 4 ounces of lean red meat per week.

Tip #4: Have no more than three alcoholic drinks a week for women, six to seven for men.

Tip #5: Watch your weight and your waist: The mirror tells all. Aim for a stable normal weight during your adult life.

Tip #6: Foods containing dietary fiber as well as nonfat milk, nonfat yogurt, calcium supplements, and calcium-containing plant foods, and garlic have been shown to be protective against this cancer. Be sure to also add vitamin D (see Tip #8 on page 330).

Tip #7: Don't smoke. Smoking increases your risk for two main reasons. First, inhaled or swallowed tobacco smoke transports carcinogens to the colon, and second, tobacco use can increase polyp size.

Tip #8: Discuss your family history with your doctor. Remember to mention if family members have had colon cancer or polyps (a precursor to colon cancer). Other cancers (such as stomach, liver, and bone) may also be relevant.

Tip #9: Get your vitamin D! (see Tip #8 on page 330).

Tip #10: Watch your insulin levels (See chapter 5, Watch Your Waistline). A study published in the *Journal of the National Cancer Institute* found that men who were on their way to getting diabetes were also likely to be on their way to getting colon cancer. Researchers tested blood samples from approximately 15,000 male doctors for C-peptide, a protein that indicates insulin levels. They found that men with the highest C-peptide levels (that is, the highest insulin levels) were almost three times more likely to develop colon cancer than men with the lowest C-peptide levels.

TOP 10 TIPS FOR LUNG CANCER PREVENTION

Tip #1: Don't smoke. Enough said.

Tip #2: If you do smoke, stop. Quitting reduces your risk of developing lung cancer, even if you've smoked for years. Talk to your health-care professional about ways to stop. Everyone knows it's difficult, but there are strategies, medications, and stop-smoking aids that can help you quit.

Tip #3: Avoid secondhand smoke. If you live or work with someone who smokes, urge him or her to quit. That doesn't always work, so the next best option is to ask them to smoke outside. Create smoke-free areas as much as possible.

Tip #4: If you do smoke, know that the combination of cigarettes, beta-carotene supplements, and alcohol is highly conducive for lung cancer development. So are cigarettes, beta-carotene supplements, and asbestos. They're both dangerous recipes for disaster.

Tip #5: Have no more than three alcoholic drinks a week for women, six to seven for men.

Tip #6: Avoid carcinogens at work. Your employer must tell you if you're exposed to toxic chemicals at your workplace. Always follow any rules that have been set up as protective measures (such as wearing a face mask). If you do work around toxic chemicals, don't smoke, as this increases your risk of lung damage.

Tip #7: Eat plenty of fruits (absolute minimum of two servings a day) and vegetables (absolute minimum of five servings a day) with a special emphasis on beta-cryptoxanthin-rich foods (see page 260).

Tip #8: Be physically active. People who are physically active may have a 30 percent to 40 percent reduced risk of developing lung cancer. The possible link between physical activity and lung cancer is based on a few studies that have found higher rates of lung cancer among those who are physically inactive compared to those who are active, after accounting for smoking status.

Tip #9: Eat apples. Apples are an excellent source of quercetin, which has been associated with a significantly decreased risk for lung cancer. Some other sources of quercetin include:

Onions (1 cup raw)	21 mg
Cranberries (1 cup)	6.7 mg
Apples (1)	6.1 mg
Blueberries (1 cup)	4.5 mg
Celery (1 cup)	4.3 mg
Broccoli (1 cup cooked)	1.7 mg
Tomatoes (1 cup raw)	1 mg
Raspberries (1 cup)	1 mg
Strawberries (1 cup)	.9 mg
Apricots (1)	.9 mg

Tip #10: Purify your water. To decrease your potential exposure to arsenic in your drinking water, consider a reverse osmosis device or bottled water for your primary drinking and cooking water supply. Although not shown to be related to lung cancer risk, when possible choose Bisphenol A–free plastic or glass containers when buying, storing, heating, or eating your food.

Appendix
and
Bibliography

Appendix

Charts and Tests

In the nineteenth century a Belgian statistician named Adolphe Quetelet developed a formula to calculate obesity. The Quetelet Index of Obesity was obtained by dividing a person's weight by the square of his or her height. In the 1980s this formula was adopted as the Body Mass Index (BMI), which became the international standard for obesity measurement. To find your BMI, see the chart on page 340.

Find your height, then look across that row. Your BMI is at the top of the column that comes closest to your weight. Normal is between 19 and 24.

Body Mass Index (BMI)

Height	19	20	21	22	23	24	25	26	27	28	29	30	35	40
							WEIGHT							
4'10"	91	96	100	105	110	115	119	124	129	134	138	143	167	191
4'11"	94	99	104	109	114	119	124	128	133	138	143	148	173	198
5'0"	97	102	107	112	118	123	128	133	138	143	148	153	179	204
5'1"	100	106	111	116	122	127	132	137	143	148	153	158	185	211
5'2"	104	109	115	120	126	131	136	142	147	153	158	164	191	218
5'3"	107	113	118	124	130	135	141	146	152	158	163	169	197	225
5'4"	110	116	122	128	134	140	145	151	157	163	169	174	204	232
5'5"	114	120	126	132	138	144	150	156	162	168	174	180	210	240
5'6"	118	124	130	136	142	148	155	161	167	173	179	186	216	247
5'7"	121	127	134	140	146	153	159	166	172	178	185	191	223	255
5'8"	125	131	138	144	151	158	164	171	177	184	190	197	230	262
5'9"	128	135	142	149	155	162	169	176	182	189	196	203	236	270
5'10"	132	139	146	153	160	167	174	181	188	195	202	207	243	278
5'11"	136	143	150	157	165	172	179	186	193	200	208	215	250	286
6'0"	140	147	154	162	169	177	184	191	199	206	213	221	258	294
6'1"	144	151	159	166	174	182	189	197	204	212	219	227	265	302
6'2"	148	155	163	171	179	186	194	202	210	218	225	233	272	311
6'3"	152	160	168	176	184	192	200	208	216	224	232	240	279	319
6'4"	156	164	172	180	189	197	205	213	221	230	238	246	287	328

Normal   Overweight   Obese

Source: National Heart, Lung, and Blood Institute

TESTING YOUR BLOOD SUGAR LEVELS

One of the things that happens as you get older is that your body's ability to control blood sugar diminishes. So as you age, you might want to check to see that your levels are within the normal range. There are several types of tests you can take to determine your blood sugar levels.

- **Fasting Blood Sugar (FBS) Test:** Your blood sugar is tested by your doctor after you have fasted for at least eight hours. If your FBS is 100 mg/dl to 125 mg/dl, you have insulin resistance, sometimes called prediabetes. If your FBS is 126 mg/dl or above, you may have diabetes.

- **Oral Glucose Tolerance Test:** This test measures your body's response to sugar. After fasting for at least eight hours, your blood is drawn to be tested. Then you drink a sweet liquid containing glucose. A blood sample is collected after one hour has passed, and again after two hours. Normal results will show a blood sugar level of less than 140 mg/dl. If your blood sugar level is 140 mg/dl to 199 mg/dl, you may have prediabetes. If your blood sugar level is 200 mg/dl or above, you may have diabetes.

- **Random Blood Sugar Test:** This means that the doctor tests your blood at any given time, not necessarily after fasting or a certain amount of time after you've eaten. A normal random blood sugar result is lower than 100 mg/dl. If your level is between 100 mg/dl and 199 mg/dl, you may have prediabetes. If your blood sugar level is 200 mg/dl or above, you may have diabetes.

- **Glycated Hemoglobin (A1C) Test:** This test is given to people who have already been diagnosed with diabetes to gauge how well they're managing their disease. The A1C test measures the weighted average of your blood sugar levels over the past two to three months. The results show what percentage of your hemoglobin is coated with sugar (glycated). People without diabetes usually test between 4 and 6 percent. Target goals for people with diabetes have recently been lowered from 7 percent to 6.5 percent. I believe that your A1C number is one of the key markers of longevity; I now have mine measured regularly. You want to keep your A1C at the low end of the normal range.

WAIST CIRCUMFERENCE AND WAIST-TO-HIP RATIO

First, stand up and measure your waist at its narrowest point (usually just above the belly button). No cheating. Breathe out normally; don't suck in your stomach. Make sure that the tape does not push tightly into your skin. Read the measurement to find your waist circumference.

Next measure your hips at the widest point of your hip bone. Then divide your waist measurement by your hip measurement.

In inches, the formula looks like this:

$$\frac{\text{Waist circumference}}{\text{Hip circumference}}$$

A person whose waist is 36 inches and whose hips are 46 inches has a waist-to-hip ratio of 0.78.

$$\frac{36"}{46"} = 0.78$$

If you are a woman and your waist circumference is more than 35 inches and/or your waist-to-hip ratio (WHR)—known in some irreverent circles as the butt-to-belly ratio—is greater than 0.8, or if you're a man with a waist circumference of more than 40 inches and/or a WHR of more than 0.9, you have an increased risk for the development of obesity-related factors including impaired glucose tolerance, insulin resistance, type 2 diabetes, high blood pressure, cataracts, macular degeneration, high triglycerides, low HDL, high total cholesterol, some types of cancer, and inflammatory markers such as C-reactive protein.

Bibliography

For a complete list of references, go to
www.superfoodsrx.com.

Chapter 1: Genesis

Freking, Kevin. Annual Health Care Spending Expected to Double by 2017. The *San Diego Union-Tribune*. February 26, 2008. Retrieved on March 10, 2008, at www.signonsandiego .com/uniontrib/2008226/news_1n26health.html.

Manini, T.M., et al. Daily activity energy expenditure and mortality among older adults. *Journal of the American Medical Association*. 2006; 296:171–79.

Chapter 2: The SuperHealth Promise and Getting Started

Bazilian, Wendy, Steven Pratt, and Kathy Matthews. *The SuperFoods Rx Diet: Lose Weight with the Power of SuperNutrients.* New York: Rodale, 2008.

Mateljan, George. *The World's Healthiest Foods: Essential Guide for the Healthiest Way of Eating.* Seattle: George Mateljan Foundation, 2006. http://whfoods.org.

Pratt, Steven, and Kathy Matthews. *SuperFoods: Fourteen Foods That Will Change Your Life.* New York: HarperCollins, 2004.

———. *SuperFoods HealthStyle: Simple Changes to Get the*

Most Out of Life for the Rest of Your Life. New York: Harper-Collins, 2006.

Chapter 3: Step 1: Control Your Genes

Afman, L., et al. Nutrigenomics: From molecular nutrition to prevention of disease. *Journal of the American Dietetic Association.* 2006; 106:569–76.

Gillies, P.J. Preemptive nutrition of pro-inflammatory states: A nutrigenomic model. *Nutrition Reviews.* 2007; 65(12):S217–S220.

Go, V.L.W., et al. Nutrient-gene interaction: metabolic genotype-phenotype relationship. *Journal of Nutrition.* 2005; 135:S3016–20.

Hall, R.D., et al. Plant metabolomics and its potential application for human nutrition. *Journal of Plant Physiology.* 2008; 132:162–75.

Kallio, P., et al. Dietary carbohydrate modification induces alterations in gene expression in abdominal subcutaneous adipose tissue in persons with the metabolic syndrome: the FUNGENUT Study. *American Journal of Clinical Nutrition.* 2007; 85:1417–27.

Kaput, J., et al. Nutritional genomics: the next frontier in the postgenomic era. *Physiology Genomics.* 2004; 16:166–77.

Mitchell, A.E., et al. Ten-year comparison of the influence of organic and conventional crop management practices on the content of flavonoids in tomato. *Journal of Agricultural Food Chemistry.* 2007; 55:6154–59.

Mutch, D.M., et al. Nutrigenomics and nutrigenetics: the emerging faces of nutrition. *Federation of American Society for Experimental Biology Journal.* 2005; 19:1602–16.

Pagmantidis, V., et al. Supplementation of healthy volunteers with nutritionally relevant amounts of selenium increases the expression of lymphocyte protein biosynthesis genes. *American Journal of Clinical Nutrition.* 2008; 87:181–89.

Roche, H.M. Dietary lipids and gene expression. *Biochemical Society Transactions.* 2004; 32(part 6):999–1002.

Salisberg, S.L., et al. Putting your genes on a diet: the molecular effects of carbohydrates. *American Journal of Clinical Nutrition.* 2007; 85:1169–70.

Simopoulos, A.P., and L.G. Cleland, eds. World Review of Nutrition and Dietetics, vol. 92. Omega-6/Omega-3 Essential Fatty Acid Ratio: The Scientific Evidence. 2003; I–XIII.

Trujillo, E., et al. Nutrigenomics, Proteomics, Metabolomics, and the Practice of Dietetics. *Journal of the American Dietetic Association.* 2006; 206:403–13.

Weaver, C., et al. Botanicals for age-related diseases: from field to practice. *American Journal of Clinical Nutrition.* 2008; 87(Suppl):S493–97.

Whalley, L.J., et al. n-3 Fatty acid erythrocyte membrane content, APOE 4, and cognitive variation: an observational follow-up study in late adulthood. *American Journal of Clinical Nutrition.* 2008; 87:S449–54.

Chapter 4: Step 2: Become an Environmentalist and Detox Your Body

Agarwal, A., et al. The effect of cell phone usage on semen analysis in men attending infertility clinic: an observational study. *Fertility & Sterility.* 2008; 89(1):124–28.

American Heart Association. *Exposure to Air Pollution Contributes to the Development of Cardiovascular Diseases (Heart Disease and Stroke).* Retrieved on Feb. 9, 2008, from http://www.americanheart.org/presenter.jhtml?identifier=4419.

Bagchi, D., and H.G. Preuss, eds. *Phytopharmaceuticals in Cancer Chemoprevention.* New York: CRC Press, 2004.

Bao, Y., and R. Fenwick, eds. *Phytochemicals in Health and Disease.* New York: Marcel Dekker, 2004.

Barth, A., et al. A meta-analysis for neurobehavioral effects due to electromagnetic field exposure emitted by GSM mobile phones. *Occupational & Environmental Medicine.* 2008; 66(5):342–46.

Brody, J., et al. Environmental pollutants and breast cancer: epidemiologic studies. *Cancer.* 2007; 109(12 Suppl): 2667–711.

———. Environmental pollutants, diet, physical activity, body size, and breast cancer. *Cancer.* 2007; 109(12 Suppl):2627–34.

Burney, P., et al. Childhood asthma and fruit consumption. *European Respiratory Journal.* 2007; 29:1161–68.

Burros, Marian. High Mercury Levels Are Found in Tuna Sushi. *The New York Times.* Jan. 23, 2008. Retrieved online Feb. 16, 2008, at www.nytimes.com/2008/01/23/dining/23sushi .html?_r=1&ex=.

Coomb, A. Breathe easier with house plants? *National Wildlife Federation Magazine.* Feb.–March 2008. 46(2):20.

Environmental Protection Agency National Center for Environmental Assessment. Dioxins: Frequently Asked Questions. Accessed on Feb. 17, 2008, at http://www.cfsan.fda.gov/ ~lrd/dioxinqa.html.

Holgate, S.T., et al. Local genetic and environmental factors in asthma disease pathogenesis: chronicity and persistence mechanisms. *European Respiratory Journal.* 2007; 29(4):793–803.

Karinen, A., et al. Mobile phone radiation might alter protein expression in human skin. *BMC Genomics.* Retrieved online on Feb. 20, 2008, at http://www.biomedcentral.com/ 1471-2164/9/77.

Klepeis, N., et al. The national human activity pattern survery (NHAPS): a resource for assessing exposure to environmental pollutants. *Journal of Exposure Analysis and Environmental Epidemiology.* 2001; 11:231–52.

Larsen, Carl. Green Is Gold with Hew-Home Program. *San Diego Union-Tribune.* Feb. 15, 2008. Accessed on Feb. 18, 2008, at http://www.signonsandiego.com/uniontrib/20080215/.

Lonn, S. Long-term mobile phone use and brain tumor risk. *American Journal of Epidemiology,* 2005; 161:526–35.

Mannino, D.M., et al. Global burden of COPD: risk factors, prevalence, and future trends. *Lancet.* 2007; 370(9589):765–73.

Organic Gardening. Air-Cleaning Plants. Oct. 2004. Accessed on Feb. 3, 2008, at http://www.organicgardening.com/ feature/0,7518,s1-5-82-1379,00.html.

Rice, P.J., et al. Advances in pesticide environmental fate and exposure assessments. *Journal of Agriculture & Food Chemistry.* 2007; 55(14):5367–76.

Rubin, C.H., et al. Exposure to persistent organochlorines among Alaska Native women. *International Journal of Circumpolar Health.* 2001; 60:157–69.

Sadetzki, S., et al. Cellular phone use and risk of benign and malignant parotid gland tumors—a nationwide case-control study. *American Journal of Epidemiology*. 2008; 167(4):457–67.

Skidmore-Roth, L., ed. *Mosby's Handbook of Herbs & Natural Supplements*. 3rd ed. New York: Elsevier Mosby, 2006.

Chapter 5: Step 3: Watch Your Waistline—Burn Those Calories

American Heart Association. Your high blood pressure questions answered—blood pressure and exercise. March 19, 2008. Retrieved online on April 1, 2008, at http://www.americanheart.org/presenter.jhtm?.

Associated Press. Experts Stress Post-Exercise Nutrition. *USA Today*. April 18, 2004. Retrieved online April 7, 2008, at http://www.usatoday.com/news/health/2004-04-18-carbs-study_x.htm.

Bloem, C., et al. Short-term exercise improves β-cell function and insulin resistance in older people with impaired glucose tolerance. *Journal of Clinical Endocrinology and Metabolism*. 2008; 92(2):387–92.

Caspersen, C.J., et al. Epidemiology of walking and type 2 diabetes. *Medicine & Science in Sports & Exercise*. 2008; 40(7):S519–28.

Dallal, C., et al. Long-term recreational physical activity and risk of invasive and in situ breast cancer. *Archives of Internal Medicine*. 2007; 167(4):408–15.

Hawkins, V. Effect of exercise on serum sex hormones in men: a 12-month randomized trial. *Medicine & Science in Sports & Exercise*. 2008; 40(2):223–33.

Katsanos, C.K., et al. Acute effects of premeal versus postmeal exercise on postprandial hypertriglyceridemia. *Clinical Journal of Sports Medicine*. 2004; 14:33–39.

Laurin, D., et al. Physical activity and risk of cognitive impairment and dementia in elderly persons. *Archives of Neurology*. 2001; 58(3):498–504.

Lee, I.M., et al. Physical activity and coronary heart disease in women: is "no pain, no gain" passé? *Journal of the American Medical Association.* 2001; 285:1447–54.

Lee, I.M., et al. The importance of walking to public health. *Medicine & Science in Sports & Exercise.* 2008; 40(7):S512–18.

Ohio State University. A Little Music with Exercise Boosts Brain Power, Study Suggests. March 24, 2004. Retrieved April 4, 2008, from http://www.sciencedaily.com/releases/2004/03/040324071444.htm.

Onishi, Norimitsu. Japan, Seeking Trim Waists, Measures Millions. *The New York Times.* June 13, 2008. Retrieved online on June 15, 2008, at www.nytimes.com/2008/06/13/word/asia/13fat.html.

Schardt, Hennah. Give Your House an Efficiency Checkup. *National Wildlife Magazine.* June–July 2008; 46(4):20–21.

Slattgery, M.L., et al. Physical activity and colon cancer: a public health perspective. *Annals of Epidemiology.* 1997; 7:137–45.

Tufts Health and Nutrition Letter. Are You Doing All You Can to Fight Sarcopenia? Muscle Loss That Leads to Frailty in Old Age Is Not Inevitable. March 2003. Retrieved online on April 6, 2008 at http://healthletter.tufts.edu/issues/2003–03/sarcopenia.html.

Weuve, J., et al. Physical activity, including walking, and cognitive function in older women. *Journal of the American Medical Association.* 2004; 292:1454–61.

Zuniga, Janine. Fine Feathered Friends. *San Diego Union-Tribune.* Retrieved online on June 12, 2008, at http://www.singonsandiego.com/uniontrib/20080609/news_1m9fowl.html.

Chapter 6: Step 4: Control Inflammation

American Association of Sleep Medicine. The Increasing Popularity of "Snoring Rooms." Retrieved online on March 20, 2008, at http://www.aasmnet.org/Articles.aspx?id=269.

Associated Press. Graveyard shift linked to cancer risk. MSNBC. Nov. 29, 2007. Retrieved online March 21, 2008, at www.msnbc.msc.com/id/22026660.

Ayas, N.T., et al. A prospective study of sleep duration and coronary heart disease in women. *Journal of the American Medical Association*. 2003; 163:205–9.

Banks, S., et al. Behavioral and physiological consequences of sleep restriction. *Journal of Clinical Sleep Medicine*. 2007; 3(5):519–28.

Bassetti, C.L. Sleep and stroke. *Seminars in Neurology*. 2005; 25(1):19–32.

Brody, S. Blood pressure reactivity to stress is better for people who recently had penile-vaginal intercourse than for people who had other or no sexual activity. *Biological Psychology*. 2006; 71(2):214–22.

Cao, H., et al. Insulin and cinnamon polyphenols increase the amount of insulin receptor b, glucose transporter 4, and anti-inflammatory protein tristetraprolin in mouse 3T3-L1 adipocytes. *The FASEB Journal*. 2006; 20:A939.

Chilton, F.H., et al. Mechanisms by which botanical lipids affect inflammatory disorders. *American Journal of Clinical Nutrition*. 2008; 87(Suppl):S498–503.

Chiuve, S.E., et al. The association between betaine and choline intakes and the plasma concentrations of homocysteine in women. *American Journal of Clinical Nutrition*. 2007; 86:1073–81.

Craig, S. Betaine in human nutrition. *American Journal of Clinical Nutrition*. 2004; 80:539–49.

Dallman, M.F., et al. Chronic stress and obesity: A new view of "comfort" food. *Proceedings of the National Academy of Science*. 2003; 100:11696–701.

Davis, S., et al. Night shift work, light at night, and risk of breast cancer. *Journal of the National Cancer Institute*. 2001; 93(20):1557–62.

Detropoulou, P., et al. Dietary choline and betaine intakes in relation to concentrations of inflammatory markers in healthy adults: the ATTICA study. *American Journal of Clinical Nutrition*. 2008; 87:424–30.

Hublin, C., et al. Sleep and Mortality: A population-based 22-year follow-up study. *Sleep*. 2007; 30(10):1245–53.

Irwin, M. Sleep deprivation and activation of morning levels of cellular and genomic markers of inflammation. *Archives of Internal Medicine*. 2006; 166(16):1756–62.

Lakka, T., et al. Effect of exercise training on plasma levels of C-reactive protein in healthy adults: the HERITAGE Family Study. *European Heart Journal.* 2005; 26(19):2018–25.

Markus, C.R., et al. Does carbohydrate-rich, protein-poor food prevent a deterioration of mood and cognitive performance of stress-prone subjects when subjected to a stressful task? *Appetite.* 1998; 31:49–65.

Meier-Ewert, H.K., et al. Effect of sleep loss on C-reactive protein, an inflammatory marker of cardiovascular risk. *Journal of the American College of Cardiology.* 2004; 43: 678–83.

Morley, J., et al. Sarcopenia. *Journal of Laboratory and Clinical Medicine.* 2001; 137:231–43.

MSNBC. Why do we need so much sleep? Accessed online on March 13, 2008, at http://www.msnbc.msn.com/id/3076707.

Resnick, H.E., et al. Diabetes and Sleep Disturbances: Findings from the Sleep Heart Health Study. *Diabetes Care.* 2003; 26:702–8.

Spiegel, et al. Effect of sleep deprivation on response to immunization. *Journal of the American Medical Association.* 2002; 288:1471–72.

Talbert, S., et al. Short sleep duration is associated with reduced leptin, elevated ghrelin, and increased body-mass index: a population-based study. *PLoS Medicine.* 2004; 3:e62.

Van Couter, E., et al. Impact of sleep and sleep loss on neuroendocrine and metabolic function. *Hormone Research.* 2007; 67(Suppl):2–9.

Van Dongen, H.P., et al. The cumulative cost of additional wakefulness: dose-response effects on neurobehavioral functions and sleep physiology from chronic sleep restriction and total sleep deprivation. *Sleep.* 2003; 26:117–26.

Yaggi, H.K., et al. Sleep duration as a risk factor for the development of type 2 diabetes. *Diabetes Care.* 2006; 29:657–61.

Zeisel, S.H. Is there a new component of the Mediterranean diet that reduces inflammation? *American Journal of Clinical Nutrition.* 2008; 87:277–78.

Chapter 7: Step 5: Keep Up Appearances

Aguirre, R., et al. Inflammation in the vascular bed: Importance of vitamin C. *Pharmacology & Therapeutics*. 2008; 119:96–103.

BBC Science and Nature. Tomatoes and Skin Protection. Retrieved online April 16, 2008, at http://www.bbc.co.uk/sn/humanbody/truthaboutfood/young/tomatoes.shtml.

Cosgrove, M., et al. Dietary nutrient intakes and skin-aging appearance among middle-aged American women. *American Journal of Clinical Nutrition*. 2007; 86(4):1225–31.

Dietrich, T., et al. Age-dependent associations between chronic periodontitis/endendulism and risk of coronary heart disease. *Circulation*. 2008; 117:1668–74.

Funasaka, Y., et al. The depigmenting effect of alpha-tocopheryol ferulate on human melanoma cells. *British Journal of Dermatology*. 1999; 141:20.

Greenway, H., and S. Pratt. Vitamins and Micronutrients in Aging and Photoaging Skin. CRC Press. In *Vegetables, Fruits, and Herbs in Health Promotion*. Ronald Ross Watson. 2000; 109–16.

Hakim, I.A., et al. Citrus peel use is associated with reduced risk of squamous cell carcinoma of the skin. *Nutrition and Cancer*. 2000; 37(2):161–68.

———. Joint effects of citrus peel use and black tea intake on the risk of squamous cell carcinoma of the skin. *BioMed Central Dermatology*. 2001; 1:3.

Harris, G., S. Pratt, et al. Superfoods and supernutrients in nutrition of the skin in *Botanical Medicine in Clinical Practice*. R.R. Watson, ed. London: Cabi, 2003.

Hegarty, V.M., et al. Tea drinking and bone mineral density in older women. *American Journal of Clinical Nutrition*. 2000; 71:1003–7.

Heinrich, U., et al. Long-term ingestion of high flavanol coca provides photoprotection against UV-induced erhthema and improves skin condition in women. *Journal of Nutrition*. 2006: 136:1565–69.

Huh, C.H., et al. A randomized, double-blind, placebo-controlled trial of vitamin C iontophoresis in melasma. *Dermatology*. 2003; 206(4):316–20.

Kafi, R., et al. Improvement of naturally aged skin with vitamin A (Retinol). *Archives of Dermatology.* 2007; 143:606–12.

Katiyar, S., et al. Green tea and skin cancer: photoimmunology, angiogenesis and DNA repair. *Journal of Nutritional Biochemistry.* 2007; 18(5):287–96.

McKay, L., et al. A review of the bioactivity of South African herbal teas: rooibos (*Aspalathus linearis*) and honeybush (*Cyclopia internedia*). *Phytotherapy Research.* 2007; 21(1):1–16.

Michna, L., et al. Inhibitory effect of voluntary running wheel exercise on UVB-induced skin carcinogenesis in SKH-1 mice. *Carcinogenesis.* 2006; 27(10):2108–15.

Neuham, K., et al. Consumption of flavanol-rich cocoa acutely increases microcirculation in human skin. *European Journal of Nutrition.* 2007; 46(1):553–56.

Pajonk, F., et al. The effects of tea extracts on proinflammatory signaling. *BMC Medicine.* 2006; 4:28.

Pratt, S., and H.T. Greenway. Nutrition and Skin Cancer Risk Prevention in *Functional Foods & Nutraceuticals in Cancer Prevention.* R.R. Watson, ed. Ames: Iowa State Press, 2003:105–20.

Purba, M., et al. Skin wrinkling: can food make a difference? *Journal of the American College of Nutrition.* 2001; 20:71–90.

Rees, J., et al. Tea consumption and basal cell and squamous cell skin cancer: results of a case-controlled study. *Journal of the American Academy of Dermatology.* 2007; 56(5): 781–85.

Sarmicanic, M. Dentists. Retrieved online April 14, 2008, at http://www.assyrianenterprise.com/DENTIST/DENTISTS.htm.

Unlu, N.Z., et al. Carotenoid absorption from salad and salsa by humans is enhanced by the addition of avocado or avocado oil. *Journal of Nutrition.* 2005; 135(3):431–36.

Chapter 8: Step 6: Preserve Your Senses

Amersbach, G. People Who Need People. *Harvard Public Health Review 2000*. Accessed online on Feb. 26, 2008, at http://www.hsph.harvard.edu/review/review_2000/feature aging.html.

Cangemi, F.E. TOZAL Study: an open case control study of an oral antioxidant and omega-3 supplement for dry AMD. *BioMed Central Ophthalmology*. 2007; 7:3.

Chasen-Taber, L., et al. A prospective study of carotenoid and vitamin A intakes and risk of cataract extraction in U.S. women. *American Journal of Clinical Nutrition*. 1999; 70:509.

Chung, E.W.T., et al. Dietary w-3 fatty acid and fish intake in the primary prevention of age-related macular degeneration. *Archives of Ophthalmology*. 2008; 126(6):826–33.

Cigarette smoking and hearing loss—the epidemiology of hearing loss study. *Journal of the American Medical Association*. 1998; 279.

Clarke, R., et al. Low vitamin B-12 status and risk of cognitive decline in older adults. *American Journal of Clinical Nutrition*. 2007; 86:1384–91.

Cohen, G.D. *The Creative Age: Awakening Human Potential in the Second Half of Life*. New York: Quill, 2000.

———. *The Mature Mind: The Positive Power of the Aging Brain*. New York: Basic Books, 2005.

Colleen, G., et al. Mechanisms of noise-induced hearing loss indicate multiple methods of prevention. *Hearing Research*. 2007; 226(1–2):22–43.

Daniel, E. Noise and hearing loss: a review. *Journal of School Health*. 2007; 77(5):225–31.

Delacourt, C., et al. Plasma lutein and zeaxanthin and other carotenoids as modifiable risk factors for age-related maculopathy and cataract: the POLA Study. *Investigative Ophthalmology and Visual Science*. 2006; 47:2329–35.

Durga, J. Effects of folic acid supplementation on hearing in older adults. *Annals of Internal Medicine*. 2007; 146:1–9.

Durga, J., et al. Effect of 3-year folic acid supplementation on cognitive function in older adults in the FACIT trial: a randomized, double blind, controlled trial. *The Lancet*. 2007; 369(9557):208–16.

Goebles, N., and M. Soyka. Dementia associated with vitamin B_{12} deficiency. *Journal of Neuropsychiatry and Clinical Neurosciences.* 200; 12:389–94.

Greenway, H., and S. Pratt. Fruit and vegetable micronutrients in diseases of the eye. CRC Press. In *Vegetables, Fruits, and Herbs in Health Promotion.* Ronald Ross Watson. 2000.

Harris, G., S. Pratt, et al. Age-related macular degeneration in *Food and Nutrition in Disease Management.* I. Kohlstadt, ed. New York: CRC Press, 2009.

Jambazian, P.R., et al. Almonds in the diet simultaneously improve plasma alpha-tocopherol concentrations and reduce plasma lipids. *Journal of the American Dietetic Association.* 2005; 105(3):449–54.

Johnson, E.J., et al. Nutritional manipulation of primate retinas, III: effects of lutein or zeaxanthin supplementation on adipose tissue and retina of xanthophyll-free monkeys. *Investigative Ophthalmology and Visual Science.* 2005; 46:692–702.

Joseph, J.A., et al. Dopamine-induced stress signaling in COS-7 cells transfected with selectively vulnerable muscarinic subreceptor types is partially mediated via the i3 loop and antagonized by blueberry extract. *Journal of Alzheimer's Disease.* 2006; 10:423–37.

———. Fruit polyphenols and their effects on neuronal signaling and behavior in senescence. *Annals of the New York Academy of Science.* 2007; 1100:470–85.

Kang, J.H., et al. Fruit and vegetable consumption and cognitive decline in aging women. *Annals of Neurology.* 2005; 57:713–20.

Khachik, F., et al. Identification of lutein and zeaxanthin oxidation products in human and monkey retinas. *Investigative Ophthalmology.* 1997; 38:1802.

Knudtson, M.D., et al. Physical activity and the 15-year cumulative incidence of age-related macular degeneration: the Beaver Dam Eye Study. *British Journal of Ophthalmology.* 2006; 90:1461–63.

Luchsinger, J., et al. Relation of higher folate intake to lower risk of Alzheimer's disease in the elderly. *Archives of Neurology.* 2007; 64:86–92.

Lytle, M.E., et al. Exercise level and cognitive decline. The

MoVIES Project. *Alzheimer's Disease and Associated Disorders.* 2004; 63:2316–21.

McElroy, Molly. Exercise shown to reverse brain deterioration brought on by aging. News Bureau University of Illinois at Urbana-Champaign. Nov. 20, 2006. Accessed online March 08, 2008, at http://www.news.uiuc.edu/news/06/1120exercise .html.

Pfeiffer, Sacha. Some Like It Hot: How Boomers' Failing Taste Buds Are Shaping the Future of American Food. *Boston Globe.* Oct. 7, 2007. Retrieved online April 10, 2008, at http://www.boston.com/news/.

Seddon, J.M., et al. Progression of age-related macular degeneration: association with dietary fat, transunsaturated fat, nuts, and fish intake. *Archives of Ophthalmology.* 2003; 121(12):1728–37.

Snodderly, D.M. Evidence for protection against age-related macular degeneration by carotenoids and antioxidant vitamins. *American Journal of Clinical Nutrition.* 1995; 62:S1448.

Sommerburg, O., et al. Fruits and vegetables that are sources for lutein and zeaxanthin: the macula pigment in human eyes. *British Journal of Ophthalmology.* 1998: 82(8):907–10.

Tan, A.G., et al. Antioxidant nutrient intake and the long-term incidence of age-related cataract: the Blue Mountains Eye Study. *American Journal of Clinical Nutrition.* 2008; 87:1899–1905.

Thornton, J., et al. Smoking and age-related macular degeneration: a review of association. *Eye.* 2005; 19(9):935–44.

Vogel, I., et al. MP3 players and hearing loss: adolescents' perceptions of loud music and hearing conservation. *Journal of Pediatrics.* 2008; 152:400–4.

Weuve, J., et al. Physical activity, including walking, and cognitive function in older women. *Journal of the American Medical Association.* 2004; 292(12):1454–61.

Wilson, R.S., et al. Loneliness and risk of Alzheimer's disease. *Archives of General Psychiatry.* 2007; 64:234–40.

Chapter 11: All-Stars: High-Fiber and Low-Sodium Food Choices, Plus Sources of Betaine, Choline, and Potassium

USDA Database for the Choline Content of Common Foods. March 2004.

Chapter 14: Preventing the 6 Major Causes of Death

Atkinson, W., et al. Dietary and supplemental betaine: acute effects on plasma betaine and homocysteine concentrations under standard and postmethionine load conditions in healthy male subjects. *American Journal of Clinical Nutrition.* 2008; 87:577–85.

Award, A.F., and P.G. Bradford, eds. *Nutrition and Cancer Prevention.* New York: CRC Taylor & Francis, 2006.

Bertone-Johnson, E.R. Prospective studies of dietary vitamin D and breast cancer: more questions raised than answered. *Nutrition Reviews.* 2007; 65(19):459–66.

Calle, E.E., et al. Overweight, obesity, and mortality from cancer in a prospectively studied cohort of U.S. adults. *New England Journal of Medicine.* 2003; 348:1625–38.

Canene-Adams, K., et al. Combinations of tomato and broccoli enhance antitumor activity in Dunning R3327H prostate adenocarcinogens. *Cancer Research.* 2007; 67:836–43.

Cordain, L. *The Paleo Diet: Lose Weight and Get Healthy by Eating the Food You Were Designed to Eat.* New York: John Wiley & Sons, 2002.

Deckelbaum, R.J., et al. Conclusions and recommendations from the symposium Beyond Cholesterol: prevention and treatment of coronary heart disease with n-3 fatty acids. *American Journal of Clinical Nutrition.* 2008;87(Suppl):S2010–12.

Delgado-Lista, J., et al. Chronic dietary fat intake modifies the postprandial response of hemostatic markers to a single fatty test meal. *American Journal of Clinical Nutrition.* 2008; 87:317–22.

Detopoulou, P., et al. Dietary choline and betaine intakes in relation to concentrations of inflammatory markers in health adults: the ATTIXCA Study. *American Journal of Clinical Nutrition.* 2008; 87:424–30.

Duffy, C., et al. Implications of phytoestrogen for breast cancer. *CA Cancer Journal for Clinicians*. 2007; 57:260–77.

Erlund, I., et al. Favorable effects of berry consumption on platelet function, blood pressure, and HDL cholesterol. *American Journal of Clinical Nutrition*. 2008; 87:323–31.

Fraser, G.E. *Diet, Life Expectancy, and Chronic Disease: Studies of Seventh-Day Adventists and Other Vegetarians*. New York: Oxford University Press, 2003.

Gnagnarella, P., et al. Glycemic index, glycemic load, and cancer risk: a meta-analysis. *American Journal of Clinical Nutrition*. 2008; 87:1793–1801.

Gronberg, H. Prostate cancer epidemiology. *Lancet*. 2003; 361:859–64.

Heilbrun, L.K., et al. Black tea consumption and cancer risk: a prospective study. *British Journal of Cancer*. 1986; 54:677–83 and L. Jian, et al. Protective effect of green tea against prostate cancer: a case-control study in southeast China. *International Journal of Cancer*. 2004; 108:130–35.

Higdon, J. *An Evidence-Based Approach to Dietary Phytochemicals*. New York: Thieme, 2007.

Houston, M.C., et al. *Hypertensive Handbook for Clinicians and Students: Pathophysiology, Diagnosis, Clinical Trials, Non Drug and Drug Treatments*. 1st ed. Birmingham, AL: ANA Publishing, 2001.

Hozaza, A., et al. Relationships of circulating carotenoids, carotenoid concentrations with several markers of inflammation, oxidative stress, and endothelial dysfunction: the Coronary Artery Risk Development in Young Adults (CARDIA) Young Adult Longitudinal Trends in Antioxidants—(YALTA) Study. *Clinical Chemistry*. 2007; 53:447–55.

Jacobson, T.A. Secondary prevention of coronary artery disease with omega-3 fatty acids. *American Journal of Cardiology*. 2006; 98(Suppl):61i–70i.

Key, T.J., et al. Plasma carotenoids, retinol, and tocopherols and the risk of prostate cancer in the European Prospective Investigation into Cancer and Nutrition Study. *American Journal of Clinical Nutrition*. 2007; 86:672–81.

Leitzmann, F., et al. Ejaculation frequency and subsequent risk of prostate cancer. *Journal of the American Medical Association*. 2004; 291:1578–86.

Lopez-Garcia, E., et al. Sleep duration, general and abdominal obesity, and weight change among the older adult population of Spain. *American Journal of Clinical Nutrition.* 2008; 87:310–16.

Ma, J., et al. A prospective study of plasma C-peptide and colorectal cancer in men. *Journal of the National Cancer Institute.* 2004; 96(7):546–53.

Malik, V., et al. Dietary prevention of atherosclerosis: go with the grains. *American Journal of Clinical Nutrition.* 2007; 85:1444–45.

Mannisto, S., et al. Dietary carotenoids and risk of lung cancer in a pooled analysis of seven cohort studies. *Cancer Epidemiology, Biomarkers and Prevention.* 2004; 13:40–48.

Manson, J. E., et al. A prospective study of walking as compared with vigorous exercises in the prevention of coronary heart disease in women. *New England Journal of Medicine.* 1999; 341:650–58.

Mellen, P.B., et al. Whole-grain intake and carotid artery atherosclerosis in a multiethnic cohort: the Insulin Resistance Atherosclerosis Study. *American Journal of Clinical Nutrition.* 2007; 85:495–502.

Nagata, Y., et al. Dietary isoflavones may protect against prostate cancer in Japanese men. *Journal Nutrition.* 2007; 137:1974–79.

Ornish, D., et al. Intensive lifestyle changes may affect the progression of prostate cancer. *Journal of Urology.* 2005; 174(3):1065–80.

Osganian, S.K., et al. Dietary carotenoids and risk of coronary artery disease in women. *American Journal of Clinical Nutrition.* 2003; 77:1390–99.

Reddy, B.S., et al. Novel approaches for colon cancer prevention by types of dietary fat, pterostilbene and other food components. Abstract AGFC 009. American Chemical Society 233rd national meeting, March 25, 2007. Accessed online March 25, 2008, at http://membership.acs.org/a/agfd/cornucopia/Spring 2007.pdf.

Rizzo, N.S., et al. Associations between physical activity, body fat, and insulin resistance (homeostasis model assessment) in adolescents: the European Youth Heart Study. *American Journal of Clinical Nutrition.* 2008; 87:586–92.

Ruano, J., et al. Intake of phenol-rich virgin olive oil improves the postprandial prothrombotic profile in hypercholesterolemic patients. *American Journal of Clinical Nutrition*. 2007; 86:341–46

Schatzkin, A., et al. Dietary fiber and whole-grain consumption in relation to colorectal cancer in the NIH-AARP Diet and Health Study. *American Journal of Clinical Nutrition*. 2007; 85:1353–60.

Spence, J.D. Homocysteine-lowering therapy: a role in stroke prevention? *Lancet Neurology*. 2007; 6:830–38.

Thompson, H., et al. In vivo investigation of changes in biomarkers of oxidative stress induced by plant food rich diets. *Journal of Agriculture, Food, and Chemistry*. 2005; 53:6126–32.

Thune, I., et al. The influence of physical activity on lung cancer risk. *International Journal of Cancer*. 1997; 70:57–62.

von Schacky, C., et al. Cardiovascular benefits of omega-3 fatty acids. *Cardiovascular Research*. 2007; 73:310–15.

Wang, L., et al. Whole- and refined-grain intakes and the risk of hypertension in women. *American Journal of Clinical Nutrition*. 2007; 86:472–79.

WHO. *World Health Statistics 2006*. Geneva, Switzerland: World Health Organization, 2006.

World Cancer Research Fund and the American Institute for Cancer Research. *Food, Nutrition, Physical Activity, and the Prevention of Cancer: A Global Perspective*. 2007. http://www.dietandcancerreport.com.

Zhang, H., et al. Blood pressure lowering for primary and secondary prevention of stroke. *Hypertension*. 2006; 48:187–95.

Index